Keeping Boundaries

Maintaining Safety and Integrity in the Psychotherapeutic Process

Keeping Boundaries

Maintaining Safety and Integrity in the Psychotherapeutic Process

Richard S. Epstein, M.D.

Clinical Professor
Department of Psychiatry
Georgetown University School of Medicine
Washington, DC

Clinical Associate Professor
Department of Psychiatry
Uniformed Services University of the Health Sciences
F. Edward Hébert School of Medicine
Bethesda, Maryland

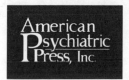

American
Psychiatric
Press, Inc.

Washington, DC
London, England

Note: The author has worked to ensure that all information in this book concerning drug dosages, schedules, and routes of administration is accurate as of the time of publication and consistent with standards set by the U.S. Food and Drug Administration and the general medical community. As medical research and practice advance, however, therapeutic standards may change. For this reason and because human and mechanical errors sometimes occur, it is recommended that readers follow the advice of a physician who is directly involved in their care or the care of a member of their family.

Books published by the American Psychiatric Press, Inc., represent the views and opinions of the individual authors and do not necessarily represent the policies and opinions of the Press or the American Psychiatric Association.

Copyright © 1994 Richard S. Epstein, M.D.
ALL RIGHTS RESERVED
Manufactured in the United States of America on acid-free paper
97 96 95 94   4 3 2 1
First Edition

American Psychiatric Press, Inc.
1400 K Street, N.W., Washington, DC 20005

Library of Congress Cataloging-in-Publication Data
Epstein, Richard S.
    Keeping boundaries: maintaining safety and integrity in the psychotherapeutic process / Richard S. Epstein. — 1st ed.
        p.   cm.
    Includes bibliographical references and index.
    ISBN 0-88048-660-0 (alk. paper)
    1. Psychotherapist and patient. 2. Psychotherapy—Moral and ethical aspects. I. Title.
    [DNLM: 1. Psychotherapy—methods. 2. Professional-Patient Relations. 3. Ethics, Medical. WM 62 E64k 1994]
RC480.8.E67 1994
616.89'14—dc20
DNLM/DLC   93-28361
for Library of Congress   CIP

British Library Cataloguing in Publication Data
A CIP record is available from the British Library.

To my teachers, whose commitment, integrity, and wisdom have continued to guide me

Contents

SECTION I

General Aspects of Therapeutic Boundaries and Boundary Violations

SECTION II

Specific Boundary Issues

SECTION III

Issues Concerning the Mental Health and Training of Psychotherapists

Acknowledgments

I would like to thank the following individuals for their help in making this book possible. Dr. Robert Simon provided invaluable assistance as my coinvestigator in our survey research on therapeutic boundaries. He also lent considerable support to the daunting task of organizing the subject matter for this text. Dr. Gary Kay played a major role as a coinvestigator in our survey research on boundaries, and brought his keen expertise to the psychometric and statistical aspects of that work. Dr. Bonnie Green and Dr. John Collette gave us discerning advice during the process of analyzing and interpreting our research data. Dr. Charles Olsen helped me to gain a better understanding of the literature on shame, and of the important role this hidden affect plays in the complex boundary phenomena occurring in the consulting room. Judge Barry Schaller was kind enough to help me in researching various aspects of the law of common carriers. I also deeply appreciate Claire Reinburg and Rebecca Richters of the American Psychiatric Press editorial staff for their diligence, persistence, and sagacity in the course of preparing this manuscript for publication.

CHAPTER 1

Introduction

A Brief Review of the Problem of Boundary Violations in Psychotherapy

In recent years, mental health clinicians have been shaken by intensifying publicity in the news media about psychotherapists exposed for unethical or exploitive behavior with patients. Some of the cases are so bizarre as to evoke a sense of living in a theater of the absurd. Despite concern that a distorted portrayal of psychiatrists in the cinema serves as a misleading form of "art imitating life" (I. Schneider 1987), we have been forced to discover that "life imitating art" in each breaking news story can prove even stranger than the tales invented by Hollywood screenwriters.

Ever an optimist, I am inclined to see a constructive side to this phenomenon. Since emotional arousal is often a precursor to understanding (Frank and Frank 1991), I believe that collective dismay may lead us toward growth and self-awareness. Just as Freud's willingness to delve into his own psychopathology led him to fruitful scientific discovery, our ability to examine why psychotherapists commit boundary violations might lead us to greater psychological understanding of human relatedness.

Gutheil and Gabbard (1993) have defined boundary violations as "boundary crossings" that are injurious to patients. Unfortunately, it is not always easy to determine if a therapist has done something harmful. Certain activities might appear innocuous on the surface, yet might impair a patient's ability to feel safe in the therapist's care. For example, if a therapist becomes involved in a conflict of interest that hampers his or her ability to concentrate primarily on the

1

patient's well-being, the patient may lose confidence and trust in the treatment (see Chapter 7), and his or her chances for recovery would then be impaired. With these considerations in mind, I use the term *boundary violation* to refer to any behavior that infringes upon the primary goal of providing care, and that might harm the patient, the therapist, or the therapy itself.

Although there are many ways that a relationship can be misused, the literature has focused primarily on therapists who eroticize the treatment. Survey studies conducted between 1973 and 1986 (Gartrell et al. 1986; Holroyd and Brodsky 1977; Kardener et al. 1973; Perry 1976; Pope and Bouhoutsos 1986 [citing Forer 1980]) revealed that from 5.5% to 13.7% of male therapists admitted to engaging in sexual activity with patients. (Women practitioners were approximately three times less likely to report such behavior.) More recent surveys suggest that this rate might be diminishing. For example, Borys and Pope (1989) found that only 0.5% of surveyed psychiatrists, psychologists, and social workers admitted having sexual contact with a current patient, and that 3.9% acknowledged having such contact after termination. These studies have had serious problems with selection bias as a result of the generally high rate of nonresponse (approximately 40%–80%). Because the nonresponders may have a higher rate of abuse than the responders, it cannot be assumed that the trend toward a reduced rate of reporting sexual involvement with patients reflects an actual reduction in the number of violations. The widespread publicity about legal sanctions against offending therapists has undoubtedly made exploitive therapists more reluctant to be candid in survey questionnaires, despite assurances of anonymity.

Clinical study of sexual violation cases reveals that offending therapists usually break boundaries in a gradual way, starting with excessive personal disclosure, accepting and giving gifts, requesting favors, and meeting patients outside the office setting. Like a seduction, the behavior escalates over time until it culminates in sexual contact (R. I. Simon 1989).

Questionnaires designed to investigate less serious violations suggest that many therapists continue to have difficulty understanding the purpose and need for boundaries in psychotherapy. For example, in a recent study of 532 psychiatrists designed to validate our Exploitation Index, a self-assessment questionnaire focusing on boundary issues (see Chapter 15 and appendix), we queried respondents about their behavior with psychotherapy patients in the previous 2 years (Epstein et al. 1992). Forty-five percent of respondents acknowledged that they touched their patients (exclusive of handshake); 32% accepted patients for treatment with whom they had had previous social contact or to whom they were related; 19% reported engaging in personal relationships with patients after treatment had terminated; 17% told patients personal details of their life in order to impress them; 17% joined in activities with patients to deceive a third party such as an insurance company; 10% admitted trying to influence patients for political causes in which they [the therapists] had a personal interest; and 7% used information gleaned from patients for their own financial or personal gain. Theoretical orientation, number of years in practice, and amount of personal psychotherapy were not significantly correlated with the frequency with which respondents endorsed these activities.

We need not rely on systematic studies alone to appreciate the scope of the problem. The media regularly report stories of well-trained and often prominent mental health professionals who have been disciplined, sued, or publicly criticized for violating ethical codes of behavior. Activities implicated in these cases have included becoming sexually involved with current or former patients, engaging in sexual affairs with patients' spouses; breaching confidentiality by speaking and writing in public about famous patients after they have died; accepting large sums of money as gifts or bequests from patients; and purchasing investments based on proprietary information revealed during psychotherapy sessions. One of the most alarming aspects of some of these cases was that the violators were highly respected teachers who functioned as important role models for their students.

Impact of the Study of Trauma and Victimology on Increased Sensitivity to Exploitation in Psychotherapy

Why has such an old problem been receiving so much attention lately? Perhaps this heightened interest is a result of an increased public awareness of the hidden nature of abuse and victimization. We have learned a great deal about trauma and violation from intensive studies of the effects of childhood incest, rape, spousal abuse, and posttraumatic stress disorder (PTSD) in general.

Often, our patients have been sexually, physically, and mentally abused as children. Their impaired sense of self-esteem and profound feelings of shame are usually organized around memories of having had their personal aspirations and sense of self invalidated by primary caregivers. Their own needs and emotions were inappropriately squelched by parental demands. Such exploitation can bring out feelings of dehumanization and "soul murder" (Shengold 1974). These experiences seem to have specifically toxic effects on the psyche. Patients injured in this way during childhood appear to be particularly vulnerable to subsequent injury if exposed to therapeutic boundary violations (Kluft 1989).

In the past, patients who were sexually exploited by their psychotherapists usually suffered in silence. In recent years, however, victims of such abuse have been receiving more encouragement to report their experiences, often through the assistance of mental health professionals, advocacy groups, and media publicity. As a result, a greater comprehension exists of the devastating confusion, sense of betrayal, and loss of trust that these patients experience as a result of their psychologically dislocating experiences (Armsworth 1990; Feldman-Summers and Jones 1984; Kluft 1989; Luepker 1990).

Another factor that appears responsible for the change in public attitudes has been the increased willingness of courts to award damages for purely mental trauma. This change may be a result of the increasing number of women entering the legal profession. Feminist scholars argue that in the past, the legal system was an exclusively male domain that valued property and physical security more highly than relationships and emotional integrity (Shuman 1992). As a result of judicial and legislative innovations, prosecutors and licensing boards are more likely to weigh psychological damages per se as a factor in their investigations and proceedings.

It has become more apparent how easy it is to underestimate the extent of a victim's psychological injuries, often because of the self-cloaking nature of the avoidant symptoms of PTSD (Epstein 1993).

In addition, studies of patients with PTSD indicate that people have a tendency to deny any personal identification with the helplessness of individuals who have experienced severe trauma, and to blame the victim (Epstein 1989; Herman 1992a). For example, many people find it difficult to believe or accept the events that transpired in the interaction between a battered wife and an abusive husband, because of an intense need to disconnect themselves from the voiceless terror, shame, and helplessness endured by the exploited woman. Relatives, neighbors, police, and even mental health professionals often defend against their feelings by telling themselves that the battered wife "deserves" her fate if she is so "crazy" as to return to live with an abusive man. Sugg and Inui (1992) queried primary care physicians about their willingness to pursue evidence of domestic violence. Their study revealed that most physicians viewed this problem as a "Pandora's box" or a "can of worms" that they avoided with the proverbial "ten-foot pole." The reasons they gave for this avoidance included fear of identifying with the victim, fear of stirring up the patient's discomfort, fear of becoming involved in a situation they felt powerless to change, and fear of feeling impotent.

Herman (1992a) suggested that one explanation for this phe-nomenon is that observers who have never been subjected to the effects of chronic terror and subjugation are likely to reason that had they been in the same situation as the victim, they would have put up more of a fight. It is likely that better awareness of these issues will continue to improve diagnostic sensitivity among mental health pro-fessionals.

Changing Professional Views About Boundary Violations in Psychotherapy

Since the early 1980s, professional societies have been taking a much more aggressive position on professional boundary violations. The early years of the psychoanalytic movement witnessed a considerable tolerance of "incestuous" involvements between analysts, students, and patients (Gutheil and Gabbard 1993; Roazen 1969). Roazen (1969) and Langs (1984–1985a) pointed out that Freud repeatedly broke his own advice regarding treatment boundaries. According to reports cited by Gutheil and Gabbard (1993), Freud treated his own daughter Anna with psychoanalysis and took meals and walks with Sandor Ferenczi during the same period in time that he was analyzing him. Similarly, within the relatively small group of early psychoanalysts, principles such as anonymity and neutrality were often violated with training analysands. The timeless nature of transference was not yet fully appreciated. Posttreatment relationships between training analysts and their former analysands often became quite intimate, at times leading to marriage. To a more limited degree, this blurring of roles appeared to continue in psychoanalytic institutes that required training analysts to act simultaneously in the roles of therapist and educational monitor (Langs 1984–1985a; Szasz 1962). In recent years, the practice of having training analysts "report" to the education committee about student analysands has largely fallen by the wayside. Most local institutes in the American Psychoanalytic Association forbid this practice. "Reporting" is seldom employed today, even in the minority of institutes in which training analysts are allowed that option (Marvin Margolis, personal communication, January 5, 1993).

Blurring of therapeutic boundaries was not limited to the disciples of Freud. For example, during the late 1960s and early 1970s, Maslow's (1968) useful concept of "self-actualization" was misinterpreted as a license to "do your own thing." Treatments modeled after "self-actualizing" encounter groups often espoused limitless pleasure seeking. These methods produced many "casualties" (Yalom and Lieberman 1971).

Until fairly recently, professional societies felt powerless to take corrective action, partly because of the ambiguity of the law and partly because of the attitude of the professional community itself. For example, in the early 1970s, a local psychiatric society attempted to expel a member for admitted sexual behavior with a patient. In the discussion leading up to an unsuccessful vote for expulsion, one of the members argued, "Why should we throw him out—she [the patient] went along with it, didn't she?"

Since 1973, however, a firming-up of the ethical guidelines has occurred (Webb 1986): patient-therapist sexuality is now absolutely prohibited. Section 2, Annotation 1, of *The Principles of Medical Ethics With Annotations Especially Applicable to Psychiatry* (American Psychiatric Association 1993) states:

> The requirement that the physician conduct himself/herself with propriety in his/her profession and in all the actions of his/her life is especially important in the case of the psychiatrist because the patient tends to model his/her behavior after that of his/her psychiatrist by identification. Further, the necessary intensity of the treatment relationship may tend to activate sexual and other needs and fantasies on the part of both patient and psychiatrist, while weakening the objectivity necessary for control. Additionally, the inherent inequality in the doctor-patient relationship may lead to exploitation of the patient. Sexual activity with a current or former patient is unethical. (p. 4)

Section 4 of the same document contains a similar proscription against sexual involvement between psychiatric faculty members and students under their training.

This evolving attitude among the mental health professions has paralleled an increased understanding of the traumatic nature of sexual boundary violations. It has also been accompanied by a large number of successful malpractice cases. At least seven states have enacted legislation governing psychotherapist-patient sex (see Table 1–1).

As an example, under the Florida Statutes, it is considered a sexual battery if sexual penetration is effected upon a person who "suffers from a mental disease or defect which renders that person temporarily or permanently incapable of appraising the nature of his or her conduct" and the offender "has reason to believe this or has actual knowledge of this fact" (Fla. Stat. § 794.011, 1b [1991]).

Professional licensing boards are now active in all states to investigate allegations of patient-psychotherapist improprieties. Following a complaint, the licensing board may appoint a professional peer review committee to conduct an investigation and make recommendations.

In contrast to the earlier laissez-faire attitude that appeared to pervade the mental health community, there are new fears that a persecutory climate may expose innocent professionals to false allegations by unstable or greedy patients hoping for a financial windfall (Slovenko 1991). Although thought to be rare, false complaints are a risk that even the most ethical psychotherapist may face (Gutheil 1992; Schoener and Milgrom 1990).

Whether or not one believes that a hysterical "witch-hunt" atmosphere has overtaken us in these litigious times, it is worth considering that adversarial positions on any subject often serve to disguise the true nature of a problem. For example, now that society at large will no longer tolerate psychotherapist-patient sex, sentiment in some professional circles has swung to the opposite pole of response—i.e., "get rid of the violator, shun him or her, and let's try to forget that something like this ever happened." This attitude conceals a widespread toleration of *nonsexual* boundary violations that may be perceived by less-restrained therapists as a form of tacit permission. We may be witnessing among mental health clinicians a phenomenon similar to the "superego lacunae" that Johnson and Szurek (1952) observed in the parents of their impulsive adolescent

Table 1–1. Examples of state regulations regarding psychotherapist-patient sexual contact

Statutory requirement	States
Therapist must report sexual exploitation by a previous therapist regardless of whether patient consents to release	MN
Civil prohibition against sexual activity with patients	CA, FL, IL, WI, MN
Therapist must wait 2 years before any sexual involvement with a *former* psychotherapy patient	CA
Criminal sanctions against sexually exploitive therapists	CA, CO, FL, IA, ME, MI, MN, NH, ND, WI, WY

Note. This table is designed to give a sampling of some of the statutory regulations in effect as of 1992. It should not be construed as a complete compendium. Various state legislatures may have enacted new laws applicable to patient-therapist sexual contact.
Source. Adapted from R. I. Simon 1992b, pp. 420–421.

patients. After acting out their parents' unconscious wishes, these adolescents would be subjected to a confusing mixture of criticism and indulgence. This phenomenon represented a form of projective identification on the part of their parents, who sought to disavow any connection with the forbidden activity. In a similar vein, Pope and Bouhoutsos (1986) alluded to the "amused tolerance" exhibited by the otherwise ethical colleagues of sexually exploitive therapists. In the same way that it works in the families of wayward adolescents, professional scapegoating of aberrant psychotherapists may foster denial and obfuscation.

The theoretical and practical evolution of psychotherapeutic methods has progressed through the study of psychic development as it unfolds on the substrate of both healthy and pathological relationships. For the same reason, however painful and embarrassing the exercise may be, it is important that we study the ways that the therapist-patient relationship can become distorted. Systematic study of therapeutic boundary violations is fairly recent. Previously, it was generally accepted that training in transference and countertransference, in combination with personal psychotherapy, would enable any ethical practitioner to cope with the problem. Repeated instances in which such grounding failed to prevent serious exploitive behavior suggests that something has been lacking in the way we screen and educate our students.

The Scope and Organization of This Book

I have written this book to provide colleagues with a review of the subject of boundary maintenance. It is designed as a guidebook to alert clinicians to the factors that serve either to protect or to damage the integrity of the treatment. Because management of therapeutic boundaries is the foundation for treatment technique, I believe that improving our understanding of this subject will enable us to be better psychotherapists for our patients and better teachers for our students. An enhanced awareness of boundary issues can also help us to be more empathic with colleagues who have committed significant violations yet remain motivated to rectify their problems. It is a basic

assumption among most psychotherapists that confronting and understanding conflictual impulses reduces one's likelihood of acting
upon irrational wishes, while at the same time increasing one's opportunities for emotional growth. The same idea applies to the potential for crossing the line in therapeutic work.

In this book I have made an effort to address the following questions:

1. What is the nature and function of the therapeutic boundary,
   and what are its developmental antecedents?
2. Are there warning signs in the interpersonal process between
   therapist and patient that can reliably predict the onset of a
   serious violation before it manifests in overt behavior?
3. Are there general characteristics of boundary violations (not limited to sexual exploitation) that would help therapists to identify
   when such violations are occurring?
4. Once a psychotherapist becomes aware that he or she might be
   engaged in a boundary violation, what is the best approach to
   dealing with the problem?
5. What are the characteristics of therapists who commit serious
   boundary violations?
6. Are there educational methods that could better prepare future
   psychotherapists to handle this issue? Conversely, are there problems in the process and structure of the present educational system that may foster boundary violations?

In Section I (Chapters 2–4), I deal with general aspects of therapeutic boundaries. Chapter 2 contains a review of the nature of personal boundaries and the way they relate to the treatment situation.
Chapter 3 outlines the developmental antecedents of ego boundaries
and treatment boundaries. Chapter 4 reviews the basic characteristics
of boundary violations.

In Section II (Chapters 5–13), I address specific types of boundary issues, including assessing the risk-benefit ratio for therapeutic
methods, evaluating the stability of the treatment setting, identifying
acceptable referral sources, encouraging patient autonomy, maintaining confidentiality, establishing coherent monetary compensation

policies, maintaining anonymity, abstaining from physical or social contact that might eroticize the treatment, and managing exploitive behavior on the part of the patient.

In Section III (Chapters 14 and 15), I deal with issues concerning the therapist's personal health and professional education. Chapter 14 addresses the characteristics of therapists who appear to be at the greatest risk for violating boundaries. Chapter 15 summarizes the problem of adverse role modeling in training programs and outlines new approaches for improving the education of psychotherapists. This chapter includes advice regarding ways that therapists might augment their boundary monitoring skills through training, supervision, continuing education, personal psychotherapy, and systematic self-assessment.

Precautions Taken in This Book to Protect Confidentiality

To avoid breaching confidentiality or causing distress to patients or therapists who might recognize their own histories, I have decided not to present any direct material from my own treatment or supervisory cases. I have taken care to use fictionalized examples constructed from *composites* of actual patients and therapists. These are "typical" scenarios that do not refer to any specific individuals. For this reason, any resemblance between the fictional persons depicted in my vignettes and an actual person, living or dead, is purely coincidental.

There are a few nonfictionalized case examples in this book that I have gathered from forensic case material or from summaries of other authors' reports in the literature. In these cases, I have endeavored to protect confidentiality by disguising identifying details to a degree that would make it highly unlikely that any close friend or relative of the individuals concerned could identify them as the subject of discussion. I have also cited a few examples drawn from television shows and the news media. Because these cases have already received widespread publicity, the issue of confidentiality does not apply. Nevertheless, by downplaying specifics such as names and places, I have tried to refrain from "spreading the gossip" any further, and have focused instead on the clinical lessons to be learned from these cases.

General Aspects of Therapeutic Boundaries and Boundary Violations

The Nature and Function of Therapeutic Boundaries

Rule 20:
A player loses the point if:
(e) He or his racket (in his hand or otherwise) or anything which he wears or carries touches the net, posts, singles sticks, cord or metal cable, strap or band, or the ground within his opponent's court at anytime while the ball is in play.
Case 4. May a player jump over the net into his opponent's court while the ball is in play and not suffer penalty?
Decision: No; he loses the point. Rule 20(e).

Rules of Tennis
United States Tennis Association (1992)[*]

What Is a Boundary? An Initial Definition

The concept of personal boundaries employs a spatial metaphor that helps us to describe and define our relationships with other beings and objects in the external world. These boundaries demarcate the line where we cease and others begin. They simultaneously encompass a recognition of our own unique existence and that of another person's identity as a separate individual with his or her own distinct thoughts, feelings, and motivations. Like the borders between nations

---

[*]Printed with permission from the U.S. Tennis Association.

and neighbors, boundaries between people validate the uniqueness and individuality of others. Psychological boundaries can be represented by actual physical barriers or may exist solely as mental representations. A person's skin and the walls of a room represent actual boundaries. A person's sense of self, the sharing of work obligations in a relationship between two persons, and the courteous respect for another person's space in a public gathering are examples of mentally defined boundaries. The manner in which these limits are handled can be the decisive factor in whether feelings of trust will evolve in a relationship. For these reasons, psychotherapeutic boundaries play a critical role in determining a patient's response to treatment.

Goffman's study of social "frames" (1974) enlarged our understanding of boundaries. He defined a frame as a sociopsychological assumption that organizes meaning and involvement in relationships. At any level of human discourse, be it loving intimacy, group process, business dealings, sporting events, or theatrical productions, all of us tend to maintain a basic set of expectations that frame the feelings of coherence and reliant expectancy by which we comprehend experiences (Goffman 1974). For instance, people waiting in line to buy tickets for a movie usually form a queue. Most expect to wait their turn on a "first come, first serve" basis. If somebody cuts into the line, the others will tend to feel confused, angry, and violated. The social frame defining their expectation of fairness has been broken.

The specific assumptions framing human interactions may vary according to nationality, ethnicity, gender, and specific subgroup membership. For example, Tannen (1990) presented evidence that women tend to frame their relationships in terms of achieving intimacy and consensual belonging, whereas men tend to organize involvement by status seeking and independence from domination. Individual variation will depend on specific psychological factors. Some people bring a trusting frame that anticipates that any new relationship will be an opportunity for a friendly, cooperative, and enjoyable encounter. Others, whose frame might be considered deviant, approach involvement with a pathological expectation. As an illustration, a sadistic individual might expect closeness and excitement to be associated with a need to inflict discomfort and humiliation on the other person.

Defining Components of the Psychotherapy Frame: The Treatment Covenant and the Fiduciary Role of the Therapist

Like any other interpersonal process, every psychotherapeutic encounter has a frame that delineates the purpose and meaning of the relationship. The therapeutic frame consists of an array of socially active components, such as a recommendation from the referring source and the therapist's professional credentials. On a more fundamental level, however, the therapeutic frame is assembled from the treatment boundaries that the therapist communicates to the patient through a series of defining messages. Some of these communications are outlined explicitly, while others are nonverbal and embedded in the therapist's behavior. As a result, the operative component of the treatment frame derives its configuration from the therapist's personal and professional ego boundaries (see Chapter 3). Although a healthy frame has coherence and consistency, it must also be adaptable in a moment-to-moment way. Ideally, the therapist will be able to fine-tune the frame into an empathic, dynamic structure that is sensitive to the patient's changing needs.

Effective treatment boundaries must be permeable at the same time that they are containing. A therapist who retreats behind an impenetrable barrier will become inaccessible. Conversely, a therapist who knows no bounds will likely foster destructive acting out. Winnicott (1960a/1965) described this balance between structure and looseness by alluding to the treatment relationship as a symbolic "transitional" space that permits the patient's expressions of fantasy. It is as if the symbols themselves have a momentary flavor of reality, while not being permitted to become so real as to be dangerous. These "transitional" creations remain safely bounded by the therapist's "professional attitude."

As a professional, every psychotherapist bears the mantle of "caregiver" bound by ethics and tradition to offer comfort and healing. The contractual agreement between psychotherapist and patient goes beyond an ordinary business agreement between two parties.

Introducing the jargon term "health care provider" removes the implied solemnity of purpose of this contract and instead suggests a strictly commercial arrangement (Frank and Frank 1991). Although the patient might be bound by certain contractual obligations to the doctor, such as payment of the fee and cooperating with the therapy, by social tradition, the doctor's obligation is more aptly described as a covenant (Webb 1986). A covenant is a *sacred* promise. A symbolic ritual is often part of the agreement. For example, in the Bible story of the covenant between God and Abraham, the "sign" of the covenant was Abraham's acceptance of circumcision for himself and his descendants. By accepting the idea of holiness and moral behavior, a surgical procedure on the male genital served as an ethical reminder and a behavioral constraint.

While the symbolic rituals connected to the healing professions might seem less extreme than religious circumcision in adult men, society continues to expect a certain rite of "sacrifice" from its healers. For example, medical training entails devoting a large part of one's young adulthood to prolonged, arduous, and sometimes traumatic study. The oft-stated purpose of this lengthy preparation is to instill in young physicians an understanding of the issues of life and death and to impress upon them the enormous responsibility involved in caring for patients. As I discuss in more detail in Chapter 15, some of the harshness of medical training has been inappropriately ritualized through the systematic shaming of students. Although such practices have often been justified as part of a rite of passage, there is evidence that their effect has been antithetical to the learning of good patient care (see Chapter 15).

The therapist's role is that of a fiduciary (Frank and Frank 1991; R. I. Simon 1987). The patient's compliance with treatment requires vulnerability and trust. Patients lack the objectivity and the expert knowledge to treat themselves, and must rely on professionals with special training. Peterson (1992) emphasized that some exploitive therapists attempt to disavow this responsibility by disclaiming any disparity in the treatment relationship. They employ pseudo-egalitarianism to exculpate themselves with the excuse that the patient was a "consenting adult."

The recitation of Hippocrates' oath, dating from the 5th century

B.C., is a ceremonial way of framing the physician's fiduciary responsibilities. It is the predominant pledge recited at U.S. medical school graduations (Dickstein et al. 1991). The format of the Hippocratic oath is that of a sacred covenant containing the ethical principles of caregiving, avoiding harm, refraining from sexual exploitation of vulnerable people, and protecting confidentiality:

> I will follow that system of regimen which according to my ability and judgment, I consider for the benefit of my patients, and abstain from whatever is deleterious and mischievous ... With purity and holiness I will pass my life and practice my Art ... Into whatever houses I enter, I will go into them for the benefit of the sick, and will abstain from every voluntary act of mischief and corruption; and, further, from the seduction of females or males, of freemen and slaves. Whatever, in connection with my professional practice or not, in connection with it, I see or hear, in the life of men, which ought not to be spoken of abroad, I will not divulge, as reckoning that all such should be kept secret. (Adams 1929, pp. 278–280)

Similarly, in Maimonides' "Prayer for the Physician," the physician seeks divine guidance in placing a patient's needs above his own vanity, cupidity, or prejudice (the actual authorship of this document is in doubt, but has been attributed to Marcus Herz [1747–1803]):

> Do not allow thirst for profit, ambition for renown and admiration, to interfere with my profession, for these are the enemies of truth and of love for mankind and they can lead astray in the great task of attending to the welfare of Thy creatures. Preserve the strength of my body and of my soul that they ever be ready to cheerfully help and support rich and poor, good and bad, enemy as well as friend. In the sufferer let me see only the human being. (Rosner 1967, pp. 451–452)

According to Dickstein et al. (1991), at the graduation ceremonies of American medical schools, the following were recited: the Oath of Hippocrates (60 schools), the Declaration of Geneva (47 schools), Maimonides' Prayer for the Physician (14 schools), and the Oath of Lasagna (4 schools). These ceremonial affirmations contain the principles that medical educators seek to impart to their graduates. They constitute the social and ethical frame of what it means to be a physician. These oaths embody six underlying ethical principles (see Table 2–1).

The principle of veracity is specifically mentioned in Section 2 of *The Principles of Medical Ethics With Annotations Especially Applicable to Psychiatry* (American Psychiatric Association 1993):

> A Physician shall deal honestly with patients and colleagues, and strive to expose those physicians deficient in character or competence, or who engage in fraud or deception. (p. 4)

Truthfulness is particularly important as an issue in psychotherapy. An honest approach fosters the patient's ability to trust both the therapist and the treatment method itself. Even minor infractions in this regard may severely undermine a patient's ability to benefit from the process.

Adverse Consequences of Pathologically Configured Treatment Frames

The suspension of critical faculties has a powerful nonspecific healing potential. This technique forms the basis for the placebo effect and hypnosis. Its manifestation in psychotherapy is the transference cure

Table 2–1. Six basic principles of medical ethics

Principle	Description
Beneficence	Applying one's abilities solely for the patient's well-being
Nonmalfeasance	Avoiding harm to the patient
Autonomy	Respecting the patient's independence
Justice	Avoiding prejudicial bias based on idiosyncrasies of the patient's background, behavior, or station in life
Confidentiality	Respecting the patient's privacy
Veracity	Maintaining truthfulness with oneself and one's patients

and the relief obtained from a supportive relationship. As with any potent medicine, there are risks as well as benefits. A powerful therapeutic agent may injure or even kill the patient. It is not uncommon for a patient's life to be literally in the therapist's hands. Because much of psychotherapy is conducted without external witnesses, the patient is extremely vulnerable to an aberrant therapist.

Patients who have been sexually exploited by their psychotherapists may react in way that is similar to childhood incest victims (Luepker 1990). Children are willing to go to almost any lengths to avoid acknowledging to themselves that the objects of their trust have deceived or hurt them. They will blame themselves rather than believe that their parents were abusive. This response relates in part to the child's self-orientation and the need to reframe any issue as something he or she can control (i.e., "They do this because I am bad; I must have deserved this pain"). Another factor is the parents' inability to admit to the destructive aspects of their behavior. Such parents often compound the injury with a blaming message that serves to justify their aberrant behavior. Regardless of his or her chronological age, a patient who has been violated by a therapist is in a dilemma similar to that of a child abuse victim. A vital frame of meaning and involvement has been shattered.

Goffman (1974) illustrated the way in which a break in the social frame can induce intense negative affects or "flooding out." A benign example would be the intense and sometimes uncontrollable laughter experienced when someone cracks a joke during a very solemn occasion such as a funeral. A break in the expected frame can be used in a theatrical production to shake up an audience or intensify their involvement. For example, one of the actors might suddenly walk off the stage and start to criticize the audience for its lack of sensitivity to a specific social issue. Psychotherapy may create an intentional break in the patient's internalized frame when the therapist refuses to accommodate an illegal request.

Some well-established social frames may be psychologically damaging. Such frames are loosely described nowadays as "dysfunctional" systems. For example, Wynne et al. (1958) described the way that families with a schizophrenic member are often structured so as to maintain an atmosphere of "pseudomutuality." In these families, members must suppress the expression of individual choice because it creates separation anxiety in the others. As a social unit, such families develop what Wynne et al. (1958) termed a *rubber fence*—an "unstable but continuous boundary with no recognizable openings" that encompasses the family system. Family members labor under the perception that this elastic boundary will fulfill all of their emotional needs. "Pseudomutuality" is seen in many other situations and is not restricted to the families of patients with schizophrenia. The seductive web of this kind of pathological frame is commonly employed by therapists who break boundaries. Outwardly, such a frame may resemble caring and friendliness. In reality, it tends to foster dependency and regressive thinking.

Because of the importance that frames play in organizing human experience, violations of treatment boundaries are likely to injure a patient's ability to hold on to a sense of meaning and involvement in relationships. People who seek treatment for mental distress have the natural expectation that the therapist will be a person who is trustworthy and stable. A therapist is supposed to be someone who is mentally healthy and able to behave rationally. Discovering that the therapist is a disturbed, dishonest, or exploitive person can be devastating to a patient.

It is possible to conceptualize the replacement of a therapeutic frame with a deviant one as a type of nightmarish transformation. This scenario is similar to an underlying theme of many horror movies, in which a good object turns into a bad object. For example, a benign and lovable thing like a cute little kitten might suddenly change into an evil and destructive monster. This phenomenon is illustrated clinically by the case of one patient who settled out of court with her elderly psychiatrist after accusing him of raping her during an Amytal interview. She described the good-object–to–bad-object transformation as follows:

> It's not supposed to happen this way! It's just not supposed to happen this way! Psychiatrists are supposed to be kindly old men who take care of you and help you solve your problems, and show you that there is good in the world! (Verbatim quotation of a guest on the Phil Donahue Show, NBC-TV, October 20, 1992)

The puzzling but serious psychopathology observed in victims of therapeutic boundary violations can be better understood from this perspective. These patients' experiences are inherently discombobulating and mind numbing. Theirs is the type of traumatic disruption experienced by people trapped inside a collapsed building or by victims of violent crimes. Their reliant expectancy of social meaning and safety has been unexpectedly violated (Epstein 1989; Shaw 1987).

General Guidelines in the Literature Regarding Coherent Treatment Boundaries

Sigmund Freud (1912/1958, 1913/1958, 1915/1958) provided specific advice about the optimal way of structuring treatment during psychoanalysis. His recommendations were based on his keen awareness of the dangers involved in analysis and the need for proper safeguards. Many of Freud's ideas remain applicable to all forms of psychotherapy. Especially relevant is his portrayal of treatment as a *container* for the patient's illness. It is easy to imagine that he was thinking of a bomb chamber when he discussed the hazards of erotic transference and countertransference:

> The psycho-analyst knows that he is working with highly explosive forces and that he needs to proceed with as much caution and conscientiousness as a chemist. But when have chemists ever been forbidden, because of the danger, from handling explosive substances, which are indispensable, on account of their effects? (Freud 1915/1958, pp. 170–171)

Freud argued that his guidelines were necessary for maintaining a reliable, trustworthy, and successful therapy, as well as for the therapist's own self-protection (Freud 1912/1958, 1913/1958, 1915/1958). Some of his advice to psychoanalysts forms the foundation of our present-day views about treatment boundaries:

1. *Informed consent*—The therapist should tell the patient about the nature of the treatment and the uncertainty of its expected duration (Freud 1913/1958).

2. *Abstinence and nonexploitation of the patient*—The patient's transference should not be confused with reality. The patient's "love" should not be exploited (Freud 1915/1958). Psychoanalysis should not be mixed with standard medical treatments. Patients should be referred to other colleagues when they require medical or surgical procedures (Freud 1913/1958). Misguided efforts to gratify the patient are likely to backfire (Freud 1919/1958).

3. *Neutrality*—The therapist's fundamental posture should be one of "sympathetic understanding." He or she should eschew the tendency to moralize, or to become an "advocate" for one side or the other if the patient happens to be in a dispute with another person (Freud 1913/1958). Similarly, the therapist should refrain from taking sides in the patient's internalized conflicts. He or she should not try to plan the patient's life by suggesting ways of sublimating primitive urges into more socially acceptable forms of expression. Such tasks should be left to the patient (Freud 1912/1958).

4. *Avoiding dual agency*—For example, the therapist should not start writing up a case for scientific publication while the patient is still in treatment, since this might tend to bring in presuppositions that will affect the therapist's unbiased listening (Freud 1912/1958). The therapist should avoid accepting a patient who may be involved in the therapist's personal or family sphere (Freud 1913/1958).

5. *Relative anonymity*—The therapist should refrain from exposing his or her own mental problems or the details of his or her intimate life to the patient in order to try to place himself or herself on a spuriously "equal footing" with the patient (Freud 1912/1958).

6. *Coherent and rational fees*—The therapist's time should be "leased." To avoid feeding into the patient's unconscious conflicts and to protect the therapist's own livelihood, the patient should be held responsible for that time even when he or she misses an appointment (Freud 1913/1958). For the same reasons, the patient should be expected to pay the fee at regular intervals (e.g., monthly). The bill should not be allowed to build up (Freud 1913/1958).

R. I. Simon (1992a) recently reviewed 11 essential boundary guidelines that he believed were necessary to maintain the integrity of treatment. Table 2–2 summarizes his inventory of recommendations for therapists.

Bleger (1966) conceptualized the therapeutic boundaries as forming a frame that is actively maintained by the therapist. On an unconscious level, the therapeutic frame is usually perceived by the patient as that which is not-self, or "non-ego." It is based on an unspoken assumption about the way things are. Only when it stops functioning does the frame become an issue. Like the ground we walk upon, we usually take no notice of it unless it suddenly fails to be there to support us. Psychotherapy patients bring into the treatment their own personal frames, which may or may not correspond with the rational boundaries actively maintained by the therapist. A patient's concealed agenda may represent a combination of rational and infantile expectations that reflect his or her core sense of discontent and concern. For example, a patient might have an assumption that the therapist will restore the lost security of childhood or that he

Table 2–2. Inventory of boundary guidelines for psychotherapists

- Obtain informed consent for all treatment procedures.
- Guard against any previous, current, or future *personal* relationship with patients.
- Arrange a stable policy regarding payment of fees.
- Provide a consistent, private, and professional setting.
- Establish a time and duration for sessions.
- Interact with patients primarily at the verbal level.
- Keep physical contact to a minimum.
- Maintain relative anonymity.
- Maintain relative neutrality.
- Encourage the patient's psychological independence.
- Protect the patient's confidentiality.

Source. Adapted from R. I. Simon 1992a.

or she will resurrect the patient's experience of omnipotent control in a symbiotic relationship.

Whatever level of reality is embedded in these longings, they usually materialize as transference phenomena in the treatment. Bleger (1966) viewed the patient's hidden agenda as a manifestation of the wish for primitive fusion with the mother of infancy. The therapeutic frame is necessary to restore enough of the feeling of symbiosis and care to enable the patient to be able to deal with his or her sense of injury. Bleger cautioned that any rupture of the realistically configured treatment frame endangered the therapeutic process. Only within a reliable and relatively unambiguous environment can the intensely irrational aspects of a patient's longings and conflicts be dealt with.

A therapist may also employ a hidden frame that contains elements highly antithetical to the overtly expressed treatment frame. He or she may not be conscious of this pathological agenda. For example, a male therapist may consciously believe that he is helping his attractive female patient to achieve autonomy by encouraging her to divorce her "loutish" and domineering husband. However, if this therapist does not help his patient to understand the nature of her dependent attachment to her husband, he may be unwittingly offering himself as a substitute authority figure in a way that will hinder his patient's growth.

Employing Bleger's terminology, Langs (1984–1985b) emphasized that maintaining the therapeutic frame was the essential core of the treatment relationship. In his view, reliably applied ground rules for psychotherapy constitute a basic form of communication to the patient about the role of the therapist, the role of the patient, and the nature of the treatment process. Thus, the therapeutic frame represents a fundamental statement about the therapist's integrity, honesty, and commitment to the patient's well-being. It demonstrates to the patient that the therapist is an organized and trustworthy person who has sufficient control over his or her own irrationality. As the result, a safe environment is created in which the patient may deal with the inherent risk of exposing his or her own primitive nature. A reliable frame represents a form of "holding" that enhances the patients's ego development and sense of both self and reality. A healthy and secure treatment frame is founded on reducing variability and uncertainty in the treatment setting as much as possible. It includes factors such as time, place, and compensation for the treatment. Sessions are held in the same setting, at a regular time of fixed duration and frequency, and for a set fee. In psychoanalytically oriented psychotherapy, the patient is responsible for paying for all sessions at which the therapist is present. The patient is instructed on free association and the therapist listens empathically with free-floating attention. The therapist avoids physical contact and maintains total confidentiality, privacy, anonymity, and neutrality.

Langs (1984–1985b) cautioned that an insecure or "deviant" frame creates a sense of confusion and mistrust in the patient. Patients often respond to boundary violations with dreams and free associations portraying the therapist as an unreliable lunatic who selfishly seeks gratification at the patient's expense. Conversely, when the therapist allows or fosters violations of the treatment frame, some patients may derive a perverse gratification that results in symptomatic relief. This temporary improvement is based on a pathological sense of victory and specialness rather than upon the patient's having achieved an enhanced sense of autonomy or self-understanding. Such an improvement is tied to a collusion with the therapist that is likely to increase dependence on whatever irrational message is being transmitted.

Langs (1984–1985b) postulated that both patient and therapist paradoxically experience phobic anxiety if the frame is secure. From the patient's point of view, a secure framework is fearfully perceived as a constraining enclosure that permits the unfolding of madness and irrationality. A therapy with leaky boundaries has a certain unconscious appeal. Such a frame makes it easier for both therapist and patient to avoid anxiety-provoking aspects of working on the problem.

Although Saari (1987) credited Lang's concept of the therapeutic frame for sensitizing therapists to the importance of monitoring the treatment environment, she faulted his views as being too inflexible. She did not believe that a statically maintained frame was necessary to protect patients from the toxic effects of the therapist. Saari argued that the therapist might become trapped in a matrix that could impair his or her ability to adapt to the patient's shifting needs. Similarly,

Palombo (1987) worried that reliance on the frame concept might lead to maladaptive blaming of therapists for their "deviant conduct." He believed that overemphasizing the therapeutic structure distracted from efforts to understand the meaning of behaviors that arise during the psychotherapeutic process.

It is important to remember that perturbations of boundaries are likely to occur even when the treatment is conducted by highly organized, ethical, and well-intentioned therapists. Nevertheless, issues such as scheduling errors, billing mistakes, and unintended contact with third parties can have a strong unconscious effect on the patient's ability to trust the therapist. One need not be a perfect therapist "machined to 15-point precision" to conduct successful treatment. Indeed, it requires a certain megalomania to believe that such perfection is attainable. What is crucial is that the therapist listen for the patient's conscious or unconscious reactions to such deviations and be prepared to understand and take responsibility for remedial action.

The therapist's role of keeping boundaries is best seen as a working paradigm, like navigating a boat by compass. Although it is impossible to be pointed in exactly the correct direction at all times, by continually observing the changes in heading, one can steer the boat back onto the proper course. Winnicott's (1960b/1965) concept of "good enough" caregiving can be usefully employed in this context. It is not necessary to be a perfect therapist, just one who is "good enough." The good-enough therapist will be able to detect and respond to the patient's spontaneous productions and gestures. As a result, the patient is able to experience the sense of validation expressed by the following statement:

> You [my therapist] appear to be influenced by what I say to you . . .
> what comes out of me has impact . . . therefore I exist as a being
> with impact and importance in the world.

The idea of being a good-enough therapist is also useful as a sobering device to quell obsessional and perfectionist strivings, even when it comes to keeping boundaries. The purpose of a well-configured therapeutic frame is to help the patient get better, not to create a jewel-studded mirror of one's own flawless technique. A therapist who is overly invested in perfection is at greater risk to impose his or her narcissistic needs upon the patient.

Keeping Boundaries as a Crucial Aspect of the Healing Process in All Treatment Modalities

Although boundary issues are rooted in psychoanalysis, their applicability is not limited to psychodynamic treatment. Psychoanalytically oriented therapists employ direct interpretation of transference phenomena with their patients. Because this approach may foster temporary regression, these clinicians probably have a greater responsibility to monitor the more subtle aspects of treatment boundaries. This does not mean that the issue should be ignored by therapists who employ a cognitive or behavioral approach. Transference regressions can occur regardless of the treatment paradigm. Patients seeking help of any kind often suspend their critical judgment in a manner quite similar to that of subjects entering a hypnotic trance.

Regardless of its therapeutic orientation, successful therapy is founded on establishing a trusting relationship. Frank and Frank (1991) reviewed evidence suggesting that all psychotherapeutic methods effect a recovery by reducing demoralization through the operation of four basic mechanisms:

1. The patient is able to establish an emotionally arousing, confidential, and trusting relationship with an individual helper (or group).
2. A structured setting is formed that is associated with the healing process.
3. A reasoned treatment method is proposed that explains the patient's problems in a plausible way and offers a ceremony or program that is intended to alleviate the symptoms.
4. The patient and therapist actively work together in the treatment program. Both believe that it will help the patient.

Similarly, Karasu (1986) considered the nonspecific aspects of change that appeared common to all therapeutic modalities. Treatments that promoted affective experiencing, cognitive mastery, and behavioral regulation appeared to be effective. The therapist's theoretical orientation did not seem to be as important as the need to have some method that fostered his or her own confidence and professional identity.

From an ethical and historical perspective, Dyer (1988) emphasized that the physician's ability to inspire the patient's trust and confidence was particularly important in ancient times, when very few treatments existed that had any specific efficacy. Despite tremendous advances in treatment methodologies, therapists must still confront clinical problems that surpass the limits of scientific knowledge. In such situations, the therapist's ability to faithfully maintain the professional role may be the only thing protecting the patient from succumbing to despair.

As is apparent from these descriptions, the common ingredients of all psychotherapies provide a structuring frame that defines meaning and involvement for the patient and enables him or her to contend with the ambiguity and uncertainty of mental distress. As far as the frame itself is concerned, the specific nature of the treatment ceremony is less important than its integrity and acceptability within the patient's rationally based value system. It is important that the therapist believe in the procedure's efficacy in order to maintain a coherence and regularity in dealing with the patient's sense of uncertainty and mistrust.

At one level or another, the clinician's personal value system will be communicated to the patient. These values may include a belief in truthfulness, an unwillingness to be corrupted either by threats or illicit gain, a respect for the patient's autonomy, and a reverence for life. This inner value system is incorporated into the fabric of specific therapeutic techniques just as reinforcing wire is impregnated into concrete. Even if the clinician's values are never spoken aloud, they form the structure that enables the treatment to succeed.

Karasu (1986) noted that "unenlightened eclecticism . . . can foster confused therapists with marginal identities" (p. 688). Similarly, Epstein and Janowsky (1969) employed the term *pseudoeclecticism* to describe the way that psychiatrists in a clinical research setting may switch ideological modes for convenience rather than in response to the patient's treatment needs. Whatever school of treatment is employed, if it is not based on the therapist's employing honesty and a fundamental respect for the patient's individuality, it has a high risk of being ineffective or even harmful to the patient.

Clinicians may become confused at times over the fact that technical procedures that might be considered normal practice in one modality (e.g., behavior therapy) might be considered quite damaging in another (e.g., psychoanalysis). For example, it would not be considered unusual for a behavioral therapist treating obsessive-compulsive patients to accompany a patient during a certain aspect of his or her daily activities as part of a program of exposure and response-inhibition. The treatment might include going to a restaurant or to a shopping mall with the patient. Such a practice is not a boundary violation because it constitutes an integral part of a coherent treatment modality that has been explained and agreed upon from the beginning. The patient has an opportunity to give informed consent before starting and the treatment is an organized professional procedure based on solid theoretical and empirical foundations.

What about the therapist who invites his attractive female patient out to dinner 6 months after they have started psychoanalytic psychotherapy? Is he justified when he reasons that he is only treating the patient's social fears by employing tried-and-true behavioral methods? This scenario would probably constitute a serious boundary violation because it represents a departure from the therapist's original and accustomed treatment method. Even if the patient acquiesced to the "change in technique," it is a highly risky procedure in the way it is proposed, and therefore violates the principle of informed consent (see Chapter 8). It is a dishonest action because it doesn't really fit the organized process of behavior therapy.

The treatment paradigm should be matched to the patient's needs, not the therapist's. For example, Miller (1991) reasoned that patients who scored high on the Openness scale of the five-factor model of personality were likely to respond better to treatments that rely on imagination and spontaneous emotional expression, such as psychoanalysis, Jungian analysis, Gestalt therapy, and hypnotically augmented psychotherapy. He suggested that low scorers would be more amenable to cognitive-behavioral methods.

A coherent treatment frame fosters psychological health and independence in a way similar to the function of the incest taboo within family units. The cultural ban against sexual relations between children and their parents or siblings operates as a social organizer in all viable human societies. Parker (1976) conducted an extensive review of anthropological and animal studies on the subject of incest, and concluded that the taboo appeared to be a culturally determined phenomenon that was facilitated by a genetically based substrate he termed incest *avoidance*. He suggested that incest avoidance is "built into the wiring" through evolutionary selection. Its survival advantage in subhuman species appears to derive from the fact that it prompts individual organisms to discover new social interactions or terrain that are distal to the nuclear parent-sibling unit. The intense physical proximity that mammalian species require in the course of caring for their young simultaneously increases the potential for sexual arousal. Were it not for the presence of a biologically determined behavioral inhibitor such as incest avoidance, offspring would be subject to developmentally crippling interactions with their parents.

Parker (1976) hypothesized that the incest taboo developed in the social structure of early human hunter-gatherers as a more complex set of behaviors and cognitions. Prehistoric human groups that developed a cognitively formalized prohibition against incest were more likely to be protected against environmental hazards, because this form of social interaction promoted individuation, novelty seeking, and curiosity and discouraged regressive dependency. For early humans, intelligence and the ability to think and behave independently were essential requirements for survival as a species. For modern-day psychotherapists, an understanding and respect for this issue can go a long way in helping us cope with our current problems. Parker (1976) summarized the link between the incest taboo and psychological development as follows:

> Only by participating in progressively wider networks of relationships does the individual form a distinct and differentiated concept of self. Thus, the incest taboo functions importantly in boundary maintenance and identity formation, without which a cultural mode of life is not possible. (Parker 1976, p. 299)

Therapy, like child care, requires a proximity of involvement that can arouse a host of passions such as lust, greed, anger, and longing for control. Like the incest taboo, the coherent treatment frame regulates the behavioral manifestation of these emotions so as to provide a safe caregiving environment. Just as the incest taboo functions as an organizer in all societies, the need for a coherent treatment frame transcends differences among schools of psychotherapy. The spectrum of therapeutic methods can be viewed as valid alternatives for alleviating emotional suffering. Like diverse languages, cultural customs, or social attire, differing theoretical orientations are psychological organizers that provide a sense of structure, meaning, and expectant regularity to personal interactions. Coherent treatment boundaries are woven into the psychotherapeutic methods of each school in a way similar to the way that diverse cultures embed the incest taboo into their social customs. The incest taboo is a core issue from which all societies derive their cohesiveness. Meaning and trust cannot be reliably sustained in groups that shirk this principle.

Summary

In this chapter, I have stressed the importance of understanding and attending to treatment boundaries. Collectively, boundaries form a coherent frame that makes healing possible. Like the incest taboo, the treatment frame is a core issue upon which all rational therapeutic technique is based. Although it may seem at times like a peripheral detail, monitoring boundaries is as essential to psychotherapy as maintaining aseptic technique is to modern surgery. To summarize:

1. Careful observation of boundaries promotes a sense of trust and helps to protect the patient's integrity as a separate individual.
2. Well-managed boundaries help to define and protect the therapist's sense of integrity as a separate person from the patient. A therapist who is able to do this sets an example that healthy self-regard can coexist in a balanced way with regard for others.
3. Coherent boundaries ensure both the patient's and the therapist's safety, promoting a trusting and honest environment. In this set-

ting, the patient can reveal traumatic memories in a manner that limits the tendency for them to be reenacted in destructive and dangerous ways.

4. Attention to boundaries augments and hastens the therapeutic process, because frank discussion of therapist-patient conflicts inspires trust and enables a patient to feel safe enough to reveal his or her hidden distress.

5. Discussion of boundary issues can be growth promoting and self-validating for the patient. Defining boundaries is a part of delineating oneself and one's unique individuality.

6. Even in the case of psychotherapeutic approaches that deliberately avoid overt exploration of the patient's hidden conflicts or transferential issues (e.g., behavior therapy), proper boundary maintenance helps to establish the therapist as a healthy role model. This imparts the behavioral message that honesty, integrity, and respect for the worth of the individual are the most adaptive ways of coping with human problems.

CHAPTER 3

Ego Boundary Development and Its Relationship to the Therapeutic Frame

Through the Thou a man becomes I. That which confronts him comes and disappears, relational events condense, then are scattered, and in the change consciousness of the unchanging partner, of the I, grows clear, and each time stronger. To be sure, it is still seen caught in the web of the relation with the Thou, as the increasingly distinguishable feature of that which reaches out to and yet is not the Thou. But it continually breaks through with more power, till a time comes when it bursts its bonds, and the I confronts itself for a moment, separated as though it were a Thou; as quickly to take possession of itself and from then on to enter into relations in consciousness of itself.

Martin Buber, *I and Thou* (1923)

The ability of a therapist to help a patient is strongly influenced by the nature of that therapist's psychological functioning. Other factors being equal, a therapist possessed of adequate self-esteem and respect for the autonomy of others is much less likely to have problems in maintaining treatment boundaries. According to this reasoning, I think that any effort to understand the problem of therapeutic boundaries must deal with certain critical aspects of mental development that are likely to influence a psychotherapist's capacity to deal with his or her thoughts and feelings during the treatment process.

In this chapter I discuss a number of facets of ego development that relate to a therapist's ability to deal with his or her own internal issues in a healthy way while at the same time differentiating them from the patient's mental processes. I approach this subject from various points of view, including ego psychology, self psychology, affect theory, the psychology of shame, psychometric research, and cognitive development. Although certain portions of this material may seem highly theoretical, I believe that it is crucial to examine these issues if we are to develop better methods of understanding and preventing therapeutic boundary violations.

Ego Boundaries

Ego boundaries can be viewed as those parts of our mental equipment that enable us to classify things existing in the world in a contextual way, according to whether they are part of ourselves or part of the external environment. This is an important element of any understanding of the psychotherapeutic process, because our ability as therapists to maintain accurate distinctions between self and other, or between fantasy and reality, will have a major impact on whether we are capable of maintaining a coherent treatment frame. Rosenbloom (1992) referred to this aspect of clinicians' functioning in his discussion of the therapist's "work ego." We can conceptualize the treatment frame as being an extension of the therapist's ego boundaries. In practical terms, this *work ego* refers to the therapist's ability to distinguish, in a consistent and reliable way, between his or her personal needs and conflicts and those of the patient. One major objective of the therapist's training and clinical experience is to reorganize and strengthen these professional ego boundaries (see Chapter 15).

Freud (1920/1958) used the phrase "a shield against stimuli" (*reizshutz*) to describe the way the developing nervous system defends itself against external impingements. He portrayed the cerebral cortex as a specialized organ that evolved to enable the living organism to filter and process incoming excitations. The cortex also regulates the internal signals of pain and pleasure that occur as a result of any breaks in the stimulus barrier. Freud (1920/1958) theorized that "an extensive breach" in this barrier led to traumatic neurosis.

Tausk (1918/1933) introduced the concept of ego boundaries to explain the puzzling beliefs of paranoid patients. In his classic article "On the Origin of the 'Influencing Machine' in Schizophrenia," he conceived of ego boundaries as the ego's "reaction" to the outside world. He believed that ego boundaries develop during the process of "object finding," as can be observed when infants explore their own body parts. The pleasure of sucking or grasping one's own body is a way of discovering external reality. Tausk reasoned that schizophrenic patients suffer from a breakdown of their ego boundaries and as a result are unable to maintain a coherent and reliable distinction between inside and outside, self and other, or past and present. Dubovsky and Groban (1975) documented the importance of sensory phenomena for the development of ego boundaries by presenting a case study of an 18-year-old man with congenital absence of sensation. This patient suffered marked deficits in self–other differentiation.

Federn (1952) employed the concept of ego boundaries in a more detailed and systematic way, to explain a variety of puzzling mental phenomena. He portrayed the ego boundary as a shifting, dynamic membrane that maintains a person's sense of self regardless of environmental variation. Although the perception of conscious awareness changes from moment to moment, like a "spotlight on the silver screen" of passing experiences, a person's ego boundaries remain as that all-encompassing net defining an enduring sense—"I" am *still* the same "me"—regardless of wide fluctuations in mental and physical contexts. Based on clinical observations, the external ego boundary may be viewed as a container for many different ego states, each of which is delineated by its own internal boundary. Compared with the usually well-defined external boundary, internal ego boundaries are much more permeable, shifting, and overlapping. For example, school-age children develop different sets of behavioral routines and internal perceptions, depending on whether they are on the playground or in the classroom (H. H. Watkins 1993). This process leads to a child's becoming aware of a "playground self" that is experienced as distinct from his or her "classroom self." The boundaries between these two ego states are quite porous, because most children are fully aware of the transition from one state to the other and are able to employ aspects of both simultaneously. Collectively, these internal states are much more rigidly distinguished from things (e.g., strangers or inanimate objects) that the child experiences as clearly external to his or her psychological space (see Figure 3–1).

Federn (1952) emphasized that ego boundaries can expand, contract, and shift to accommodate an individual's changing emotional investments. Like an amoeba's cell membrane, the ego may change

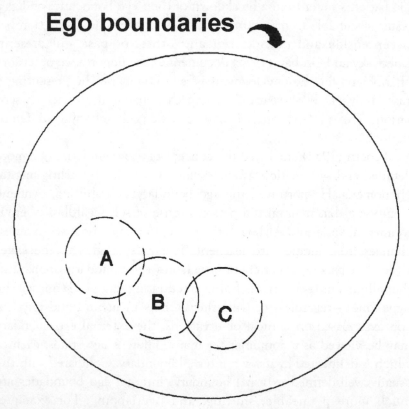

Figure 3–1. Diagrammatic conceptualization of ego boundaries in normal adults. The ego boundaries maintain an individual's encompassing and persisting sense of having a continuous "me," despite fluctuations resulting from behavioral repertoires and changes in the external environment through time and geographic location. The different ego states denoted by *dotted circles* A, B, and C represent the internal boundaries of overlapping and highly permeable states of personal experience.

shape and incorporate new objects while remaining the same entity. Subsequent authors elaborated Federn's metaphor as a way of defining and treating discretely experienced ego states encompassed within a system of external and internal boundaries (Berne 1964; Durkin 1982; Perls 1969; Szekacs 1985; H. H. Watkins 1993; J. G. Watkins and H. H. Watkins 1982, 1988, 1990; Winnicott 1960c/1965).

Berne (1964) employed the terms *child*, *parent*, and *adult* to describe the ego states that formed the foundation for his theory of Transactional Analysis. Gestalt therapy also relies heavily on the ego boundary concept to define states of being (Perls 1969). For example, in Gestalt therapy, patients might be asked to play the roles of various elements in their dreams, such as a tissue box, a ticket agent, a vicious animal, or an abusive parent. This activity allows them to identify and "reown" disavowed internalized ego states (Perls 1969).

J. G. Watkins and H. H. Watkins (1982, 1988, 1990) developed a psychotherapeutic method based on their observation that intrapsychic conflicts result from interactions among a myriad of encapsulated ego states. In most individuals, the boundaries of these internalized formations are more diffuse than those seen in the dissociated "alters" of patients with multiple personality disorder (see Figures 3–1 and 3–2).

Durkin (1982) employed von Bertalanffy's general systems theory (von Bertalanffy 1968) to study the nature of boundary formation in psychotherapy groups. Any organized biological unit, be it a single individual or a social aggregate, is able to survive only by maintaining boundaries that are permeable enough to allow for interchange with the environment. Rather than maintaining a rigid steady state, healthy living systems are able to adapt flexibly to changing circumstances while at the same time keeping their unique identity. Durkin (1982) found that pathological adaptations could be effectively treated if the therapist endeavored to open or close boundaries at various hierarchical levels of the psychotherapy group. These levels included the group itself, its individual members, and a given individual's internalized ego states.

Psychometric tests of ego boundary function have provided an opportunity to study the ego boundary concept in a systematic and

Overall "system" ego boundaries

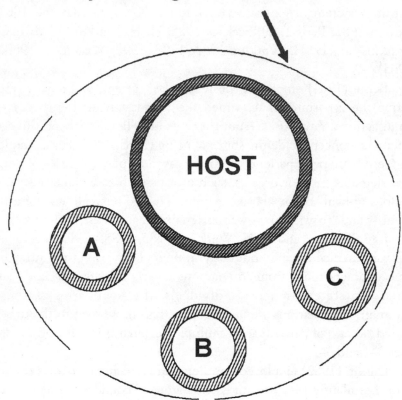

Figure 3–2. Diagrammatic conceptualization of dissociative disorders in terms of defects in internal and external ego boundaries. In patients with severe dissociative disorders such as multiple personality disorder, the external ego boundaries are very porous (*gaps in the outermost circle*). This condition often results from repeated violations of the patient's personal space during childhood (e.g., by incest or physical abuse). The pathologically thickened internal ego boundaries (*Host, A, B,* and *C*) are experienced as "alters" that defend against the pathological interruptions in the external boundaries. The ego boundaries can be likened to inner citadels of security in a besieged city whose outer walls have been breached by an enemy. In Ganser syndrome, the dissociated ego states may protect against an underlying psychosis (Epstein 1991).

quantitative way (Celenza 1986; Hartmann 1991; Lerner et al. 1985; Levin 1990; Senior 1981). For example, Lerner et al. (1985) employed the Boundary Disturbance Scale of the Rorschach to distinguish the qualitative differences in response among patients with schizophrenia, patients with borderline personality disorder, and healthy controls. Schizophrenic patients offered significantly more "contaminated" responses (i.e., gross reliance on primary process mechanisms such as condensing two unrelated concepts) than did borderline patients or controls. The authors interpreted this difference as an indication that the patients with schizophrenia had a marked impairment of their "self–other" boundaries. On the other hand, the patients with borderline personality disorder endorsed more "confabulation responses," suggesting an impairment of their "inner–outer" boundaries (i.e., they found it difficult to differentiate fantasy from reality).

Senior (1981) employed Landis's scoring of the Rorschach (Landis 1970) to assess "permeability" and "impermeability" of the external ego boundaries. She compared these scores with other psychological measures designed to assess the "firmness" of internal ego states (*internal tension regions*). Subjects with the least permeable external boundaries tended to have internalized states that were more firmly defined than those of individuals whose external boundaries were highly permeable. This trend was demonstrated by significant correlations with subscores on the Rorschach, but not by the overall external permeability scores. Senior's findings are in accord with Durkin's (1982) view, following von Bertalanffy's (1968) general systems theory, that complex systems are organized isomorphically. In other words, a superordinate system will tend to have the same functional characteristics as its component subsystems. Senior (1981) concluded that measures of boundary permeability and impermeability should be treated as separate variables, not as bipolarities of a single dimension. This point of view dovetails with the clinical observation that healthy, adaptive ego functioning requires a flexible capacity to be both open and steadfast.

The ego boundary construct would lose much of its usefulness if limited in a simplistic fashion to a spatial metaphor distinguishing inner thoughts from external reality. Rather, it is best viewed as a model for elucidating a dynamically changing, multidimensional system. In this regard, Polster (1983) cautioned against the common proclivity of psychodynamic clinicians to conceptualize the ego boundary solely in terms of its function as a strong or weak barrier between outside and inside. She argued that this perspective fails to account for the active process by which humans define their contextual relations with the world. Polster believed that it was more useful to view ego boundaries as that part of one's psyche that can maintain a sense of constancy in classifying reality (i.e., in categorizing and sequencing) and in locating oneself as an entity within the matrix of that reality. She proposed that a person's ego boundary functioning be assessed according to his or her ability to include and separate.

Celenza (1986) attempted to use measures of ego boundary functioning to distinguish empathic capacity in normal, narcissistic, and borderline subjects. Among several measures, she employed Corcoran's (1982) Maintenance of Emotional Separation (MES) scale and Hartmann's Boundary Questionnaire (BQ) as independent variables (see the detailed discussion of Hartmann's [1991] findings later in this chapter). Subjects scoring in the intermediate range on boundary measures were considered to have flexible rather than thick or thin boundaries. Celenza found that empathy was associated with boundary flexibility as measured by the MES scale but not by the BQ. The MES scale assesses self-definition by scoring the intensity with which the subject identifies with another person's distress. The BQ measures the tendency for diffuseness in both internal boundary states and self–other differentiation. In addition, most of the BQ items measure traits rather than adaptive reactions to specific interpersonal situations. Like Polster (1983), Celenza (1986) warned that use of the ego boundary construct could be very misleading, particularly when employed in its most narrow sense of self–other differentiation. Much confusion results from the fact that internal ego states based on traumatic experiences are very prone to become disconnected from conscious awareness. These states may subsequently become projected onto other individuals. Following such a projection, it becomes very difficult for either the first person (the projector) or the other person (the projectee) to determine who actually "owns" the psychic contents in question, and on which side of the "bound-

ary" the problem actually resides (see the section on projective identification later in this chapter).

Table 3–1 summarizes the construct of ego boundaries according
to the functions described in this section.

In my own clinical experience, I have found most patients readily
able to employ the boundary metaphor as an effective way of organizing their most chaotic experiences. Clinical evidence suggests that
much of the confusion that a patient experiences regarding his or her
interpersonal conflicts can be more quickly resolved if the therapist
can help the patient to address disavowed and conflict-ridden internal ego states (Berne 1964; Durkin 1982; Perls 1969; Szekacs 1985;
H. H. Watkins 1993; J. G. Watkins and H. H. Watkins 1982, 1988,
1990). Similarly, I believe that a better understanding of disconnected internal ego states can help us to explain some of the more
puzzling aspects of therapeutic boundary violations.

Table 3–1. The "ego boundary" construct defined in terms of its
hypothesized operations

Healthy ego boundaries perform the following functions:
- Perceive experiences (*Inclusion*)
- Shut out experiences (*Exclusion*)
- Include and exclude various things according to coherent categories
  (*Categorical Classification*)
- Actively process and define one's relationships with things in the
  animate and inanimate world, depending on active changes in their
  properties or behavior (*Contextual Classification*)
- Distinguish oneself from other persons (*Self–Other Differentiation*)
- Acknowledge "ownership" of one's internal states and distinguish them
  from external states (*Differentiating Symbols [Mental Processes] From
  External Reality*)
- Flexibly adapt to changing circumstances such as time, place, and
  environmental stress while simultaneously maintaining a unique identity
  (*Maintaining Identity*)
- Maintain an internal representation of oneself in conjunction with the
  images of other persons with whom one has past and ongoing
  relationships (*Monitoring Object Relationships*)
- Identify with another person's emotional state (*Empathy*)

For heuristic purposes, I have employed a series of diagrams like the one in Figure 3–1 to clarify some of the complex processes occurring in the therapeutic setting. Like a single section from a cerebral magnetic resonance imaging (MRI), a picture can be helpful even if it cannot be expected to reveal the total nature of a multidimensional, dynamic structure as it changes over time. I have pictured overly porous (thin) boundaries in my diagrams by using interrupted lines. Overly dense (thick) boundaries are denoted by a shaded region. It might have been more "physiological" to portray the dynamic adaptability of an ego boundary by depicting "gating" sites similar to the channels that regulate ion flux through cell membranes. Overly porous boundaries would result from gates that could not close sufficiently, and overly dense boundaries from those that could not open. Healthy boundaries would be flexible enough to open or close in response to ambient conditions (see Figure 3–3). A person's ego boundary may be excessively permeable in one aspect of its functioning and overly impermeable in another. Such a condition would explain Senior's (1981) finding that the two measures do not appear to exist on a bipolar continuum. Portraying this state diagrammatically would entail drawing certain segments of the ego boundary with thin gating sites and others with thick sites. For simplicity of presentation, I have elected to omit these gating sites from the figures, and to leave it to the reader to mentally insert this detail.

The presence of healthy and flexible ego boundaries accounts for the way we fragile creatures are able to maintain a continuous and coherent sense of ourselves, even in the face of horrendous environmental changes. The gating channels of our boundaries are able to adjust flexibly to internal and external conditions by opening or closing at the appropriate times. Pathological states such as psychotic regression, pathological narcissism, and depersonalization can be explained as a consequence of excessive thinning or thickening of the internal and external ego boundaries. A case of a man suffering from depersonalization illustrates this concept:

> After his 21st birthday, Mr. Aaron began to experience a progressive sense of bodily detachment and depletion. He was a large, muscular man. His father, a retired butcher, had physically abused

"Gate" position

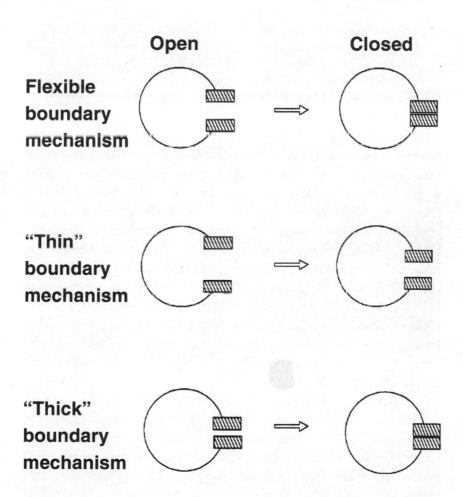

Figure 3–3. Conceptualization of ego boundary "gating" mechanisms. The *shaded rectangles* encompass channels at the surface of the ego boundary. These channels function as the "gates" that regulate the flow between the psyche and the external world. Normal gates are able to open or close flexibly, depending on the person's adaptive needs. Excessively porous boundaries are caused by an inability to close the gates sufficiently. Inordinately dense boundaries are caused by gates that cannot open sufficiently.

Mr. Aaron's mother. Mr. Aaron's symptoms began when he began to identify his developing adult body with that of his brutal and powerful father, whom he closely resembled. He could not stand "being" his father. His unconscious mind rejected the "father in-side" and his internal ego boundaries became pathologically recon-figured to exclude this traumatically disavowed aspect of himself. He was left feeling depersonalized and *weak*. Psychotherapy pro-vided relief of his symptoms as he worked through this conflicted identification (see Figure 3–4).

Healthy ego boundaries function as a gating device that dis-tinguishes between inside and outside and among internal ego states. Like any organ system maintaining homeostasis, these gates serve a regulatory function. Ideally, ego boundaries should be both permeable enough to allow information to penetrate the system and thick enough to maintain coherence. It is important to consider the stage of development and the nature of the defect in any discussion of ego boundary dysfunction. Ego boundary impairment may involve various combinations of excessive porosity and thickening. Infants have highly permeable boundaries. Retaining such a marked looseness in adult life can predispose to serious psychopathology. On the other hand, porous boundaries appear to be correlated with sensitivity and creativity. Overly dense boundaries in adult life allow for a high degree of stability but may impair an individual's ability to under-stand other people's feelings.

Let us return to the issue with which we began our discussion of ego boundaries. Organizing a proper treatment frame means that the therapist must adhere to the goal of helping the patient and must assiduously refrain from exploiting the patient's vulnerabilities. This means that the therapist must be able to maintain a consistency of purpose regardless of any distraction or temptation. He or she must also be prepared to cope with the patient's disavowed ego states, especially those that might resonate with the therapist's own internal conflicts. Such an undertaking is possible only if the therapist has achieved sufficient ability to determine, in a contextually appropriate way, the difference between what is going on inside the patient and what is going on inside himself or herself. This capacity can be seen as the essential function of the therapist's professional ego boundaries, which must be strengthened and organized though training, personal psychotherapy, and an enduring commitment to the patient's well-being.

For many patients, it is this extension of the therapist's professional boundaries that provides the critical support that permits healing to occur. Many individuals who suffer from disorganized and

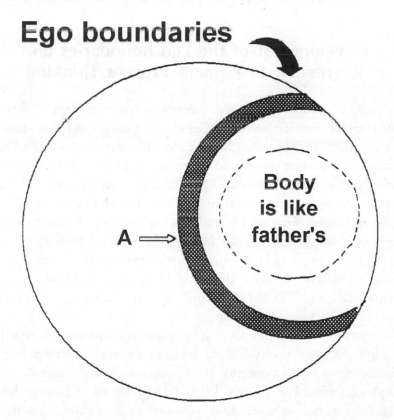

Figure 3–4. Diagrammatic conceptualization of Mr. Aaron's depersonalization in terms of the configuration of his ego boundaries. Under normal circumstances, the internalized ego state "my body is like my father's" (*dotted circle*) would have highly permeable internal boundaries in relation to the rest of his psyche. Because of his need to disavow any sense of identification with his father's physical brutality, Mr. Aaron erected a pathologically dense internal boundary (A). As a result, he was unable to perceive his body as being fully a part of himself.

maladaptive boundary configurations cannot recover without a therapist who possesses an organized and coherent set of treatment boundaries. The therapist serves as a temporary "prosthesis" that enables
these patients to safely cope with their unbearable mental contents.
In practical terms, the "prosthetic" function might be performed by
the treatment contract with the individual therapist, the cohesive
group in group psychotherapy, the "bridge graft" function of a home
care nurse (Epstein 1982), or the structure provided by hospital staff.

Development of the Ego Boundaries and Regression to Primary Process Thinking

In earliest infancy, the psychic apparatus has very little ability to
differentiate between an "inside" and an "outside." At this stage of
development, the ego boundaries enclose the universal set of all sen-
sations and are not yet able to differentiate a coherent "me" from a
coherent "not-me." They may be likened to a highly permeable, all-
encompassing membrane that envelops totality and infinitude. These
loose and highly expanded boundaries sustain a peculiar and chaotic
form of thinking that Freud (1900/1958) termed *primary process*.
Spitz (1965) employed the term *coenesthetic reception* (literally, "common feeling") to describe this form of mentation. More recently,
Matte-Blanco (1988) has elucidated some of the interesting properties of primary process thinking.

As its ego boundaries develop the capacity to distinguish an inner
me from an outer you, the child develops a corresponding ability to
classify objects and concepts in logical, linear, and rational ways,
employing what Freud (1900/1958) termed *secondary process* thinking. We can conceptualize that secondary process thinking is maintained by the filtering capacities of the ego boundaries. Primary
process thinking operates on the "pleasure principle" rather than according to the demands of reality. It is also characterized by timeless-
ness and the absence of negation or finitude. Table 3–2 summarizes
the formal characteristics of the primary process.

Even in adults with firmly established ego boundaries, primary
process thinking continues to operate as the predominant substrate of

the unconscious mind. It is observable in creative activity, dreams, fantasy, parapraxes, hypnotic trances, drug intoxication, and psychosis. At these times, the ego boundaries become extremely porous and have a diminished capacity to distinguish external from internal reality.

Primary process thinking is often consciously employed by nonpsychotic adults in a curious amalgamation with normal rational thinking. Orne (1959) coined the term *trance logic* to characterize this phenomenon, which occurs when false conclusions—based on predominantly primary process operations—are seamlessly intermixed with ordinary rational thinking in an effort to explain away impossible inconsistencies. Orne found that hypnotized subjects could be reliably distinguished from simulators by the presence of trance logic, which he defined as "the apparently simultaneous perception and response to both hallucinations and reality, without any apparent attempt to satisfy a need for logical consistency" (Orne 1959, p. 295). In his experiments, highly hypnotizable subjects were seated and placed in a trance at a time when they could plainly see a coexperimenter sitting to one side in their field of view. During the trance, the subjects were told that they would slowly open their eyes (while still hypnotized) and would see the coexperimenter sitting in the

Table 3–2. Formal characteristics of primary process thinking

- Gradations are absent—perceptions are "all or nothing."
- Perceptions are visceral and global.
- Communication is nondirected and predominantly gestural.
- Negation is lacking.
- Mutual contradictions coexist.
- Concepts are displaced onto one another.
- Two or more concepts are condensed into one.
- Time as a unidirectional and sequential flow is absent.
- Internal reality is substituted for external reality.
- Alternatives are identified as being equivalent.

Source. Adapted from Rayner and Tuckett 1988, pp. 8–9; and Spitz 1965, pp. 138–143.

same location. Unbeknownst to the subjects, the coexperimenter had quietly shifted location to a chair behind them. The subjects hallucinated an image of the coexperimenter in the first location, but commented on the peculiar fact that they could "see the chair through him," as if he were transparent. They became confused when they were then asked to turn around and describe what they saw while gazing at the real coexperimenter. Although confounded by seeing a "double" person, they were not overly upset by this experience and ascribed it to "mirrors" or a "trick" (Orne 1959). In their studies replicating Orne's findings, Marks et al. (1989) reported that their subjects experienced a sense of surprise at seeing the double, and in several instances offered quasi-rational explanations for the phenomenon, such as reasoning that the target individual had a twin brother, or that he was able to run very fast from one location to the other.

Trance logic is observed in patients with Ganser syndrome, a dissociative disorder that usually stems from a reaction to trauma (Epstein 1991). Sometimes this disorder arises as a defense against an impending psychosis. Ganser (1904) noted that his patients did not appear disturbed by the obvious inconsistency between their answers to his questions and physical reality. For example, when he asked one patient "How many ears do you have?" the patient answered "Four." Ganser attempted to pursue the logic being employed, and asked the patient to show him where they were. The patient pointed to two "outer" and two "inner" ears.

In dissociative disorders, isolated islands of self defined by rigidly compartmentalized internal ego boundaries appear to coexist without full integration with one another. This discrepant experience is maintained by use of trance logic. It is like a split-screen video that displays simultaneous but separate aspects of an event. This condition is also similar to the "splitting" of the ego that occurs in fetishism (Schafer 1968). The use of trance logic can explain much of the bizarre symptomatology seen in more chronic dissociative illnesses such as multiple personality disorder (Epstein 1991). In dissociative disorders, the external ego boundaries are damaged—as a result of traumatization and comorbid psychopathology—at the same time that the boundaries of internal ego states have become pathologically thickened (J. G. Watkins and H. H. Watkins 1988) (see Figure 3–2).

Matte-Blanco's work provides an interesting way of understanding the phenomenological aspects of trance logic and its amalgamation of rationality and irrationality (Arden 1984; Matte-Blanco 1959, 1988; Raynor and Tuckett 1988). Matte-Blanco analyzed the formal mechanisms that distinguish primary from secondary process thinking, and developed mathematical analogies based on set theory and multidimensional operations (see also Arden 1984; Raynor and Tuckett 1988). The secondary process employs what he called *asymmetrical* thinking—the foundation for Aristotelian syllogism, causal logic, and scientific understanding. "I throw the ball" is an asymmetrical statement. It doesn't mean the same thing if we exchange the subject and predicate and say "The ball throws I (me)." In a symmetrical statement, the meaning stays the same with this switch, like a grammatical palindrome. For example, "John is the sibling of Mary" has the same meaning as "Mary is the sibling of John." Matte-Blanco (1988) demonstrated how symmetrical thinking is implicit in Freud's descriptions of unconscious mentation. In dreams, for example, objects may be equated with each other even if they have only a trivial feature in common. This phenomenon is reflected in the mechanisms of condensation, displacement, and representation of a whole by one of its parts.

In secondary process thinking, two subsets of a larger set, such as apples and oranges, can be distinguished as separate categories even though they are subsets of the superordinate category of "fruit." If a person's ego boundaries are defective, his or her ability to classify reality will revert to primary process logic. An individual who cannot distinguish "I" from "not-I" will also fail in attempts to differentiate between apples and oranges. Impaired boundaries lead to impaired reasoning (see Figure 3–5).

Matte-Blanco (1988) employed the term *bilogical reasoning* to describe the various combinations of primary and secondary process thinking that both healthy and psychiatrically disturbed individuals may employ. His formulations provide a rich and detailed way of understanding and categorizing projective identification and other admixtures of rational and irrational thinking as they arise in the psychotherapeutic setting.

The terms *trance logic* and *bilogical reasoning* refer to similar phe-

A. Primary process ego boundaries

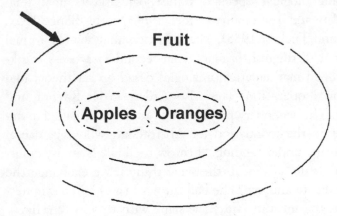

B. Secondary process ego boundaries

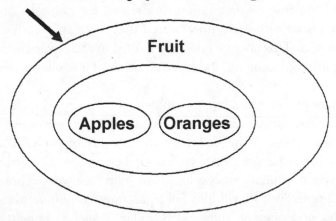

Figure 3–5. Embedded Venn diagrams showing how the ability to "classify" objects is related to the state of a person's ego boundaries. The individual in condition A uses predominantly primary process thinking. As a result, this person's ability to maintain the "boundaries" between logical concepts is impaired. Because of defects in ego boundaries, such a person is unable to reliably classify "apples" and "oranges" as different subcategories of the larger category of "fruit." The individual in condition B has ego boundaries that are intact. This person is able to maintain a crisp conceptual differentiation of the categories and their classification.

nomena. Herman (1992b) used an equivalent term derived from George Orwell's novel *1984—doublethink*. This word evokes the dissociated mentation connected with chronic terror and abuse. From a scientific standpoint, *trance logic* has the advantage of being experimentally defined and reproducible. What is so striking about Orne's (1959) experiments is the fact that the ego boundaries of highly hypnotizable subjects were artificially compartmentalized into dissociated segments. When these nonpsychotic individuals were induced to "see" things that weren't there, they rationalized the mutual inconsistencies inherent in the hallucinations by using reasoning supported mainly by primary process logic. Thus, it was demonstrated that an overly rigid compartmentalization in the ego boundaries results in defects in a person's ability to differentiate internal images from external reality.

Through suspension of critical judgment, Orne's subjects transferred a portion of their ego boundaries over to the experimenter. The experimenter's suggestions became a new, superordinate frame of reality. When an impossible reality was assigned by the experimenter (i.e., a hallucination induced by a suggested image), the defect in the subject's ego boundaries became apparent and had to be covered over by an "explanation" consisting of a patched-together amalgamation of the experimenter's impossible suggestion and the subject's more primitive ego states.

In their most extreme manifestation, archaic ego states are seen in the irrational child alters of patients with multiple personality disorder. Although they have a coherent definition, the alters are often quite detached from external reality and tend to rely on heavy doses of primary process thinking (Alpher 1991). It should be emphasized, however, that even healthy individuals are likely to possess internal ego states that to varying degrees are disconnected from full awareness.

This discussion of primary process, trance logic, and bilogical thinking can assist us in understanding some of the mechanisms of therapeutic boundary violations and in developing a better way of preventing such violations from occurring. As I review in Chapter 4, nonpsychotic and nonpsychopathic therapists can also become quite disconnected from the realities of their task. As their therapeutic ego boundaries become damaged by a variety of stressors they are unprepared to handle, they cover the gaps with an impaired ego state organized by primary process thinking cloaked in a masquerade of rationality. The occurrence of trance logic or bilogical thinking becomes an indicator of the fact that a dissociated internalized state may be operating on a semi-independent basis within the therapist.

Biological Versus Environmental Aspects of Ego Boundaries

An impairment in ego boundaries appears to be a regular feature of psychotic disorders (Tausk 1918/1933). The fact that illnesses such as schizophrenia and bipolar disorder are heritable conditions suggests that there may be a significant genetic component in an individual's capacity to maintain a coherent sense of self. Hartmann et al. (1987) studied this issue in individuals suffering from chronic nightmares. About one-third of their 12 subjects suffered from DSM-III disorders such as schizoid, schizotypal, and borderline personality disorders. One individual had schizophrenia. Regardless of the presence of psychopathology, the subjects' personalities could be characterized as "open, vulnerable, defenseless, and artistic." Their ego boundaries appeared very penetrable or "thin," as measured both clinically and by psychological testing based on the Rorschach. Hartmann (1991) developed his Boundary Questionnaire (BQ) as a means of investigating this concept in greater depth. He administered the BQ to 866 subjects and studied the characteristics of 40 individuals with the highest scores (very "thin" boundaries) and lowest scores (very "thick" boundaries). One statement that appeared to be the best identifier of an individual with thin boundaries was "I have had the experience of someone calling me or speaking my name and of not being sure whether it was really happening or I was imagining it."

Respondents with thick boundaries tended to think in a strictly linear fashion and had difficulty associating freely. They were conventional and practical-minded "live-in-the-present" types, and were likely to be employed in business, law, or engineering. Their personalities appeared to be solid, well grounded, and at times obsessional.

They viewed people with thin boundaries as being "flaky." When individuals with thick boundaries were asked to elaborate upon their feelings, they were likely to answer "Well that's it," "That's how it is," or "There's nothing more to say." (Hartmann 1991, p. 26).

Conversely, individuals with thin boundaries were able to free-associate quite readily, to such an extent that they did so in inappropriate situations. They were highly oriented to the past as well as to the present, and had a vivid perception of their memories. They were often employed as teachers, artists, and health and human services workers.

Factor analysis of Hartmann's (1991) BQ revealed that the first factor included 51 questions (of a total of 145) that addressed experiences such as merging objects with self and each other and fluctuating identity. Hartmann named this factor *primary process thinking*.

Based on his use of the BQ with both clinical and research populations, as well as on some evidence for concordance among siblings, Hartmann (1991) suggested that there is a genetic component that explains boundary permeability. He found that subjects with thin boundaries were better able to lower their skin temperature using visual imagery than were those with thick boundaries (Hartmann 1991). This capability indicated a significant correlation between hypnotic responsiveness and boundary permeability. Evidence showing a genetic component in hypnotic responsiveness (Olness and Gardner 1988) lends further support to Hartmann's hypothesis.

Hartmann (1991) employed neuropsychological testing and found that thick-boundaried individuals were more structured in their approaches to tasks. At the same time, they were more perseverative than were thin-boundaried subjects, who were less organized but more flexible in their approaches to the tests. Hartmann also cited sleep electroencephalogram (EEG) evidence for a dissociation between rapid eye movement (REM) and non-REM sleep in thin-boundaried individuals (Hartmann 1991).

In considering the environmental and developmental factors that might explain why an individual develops thick as opposed to thin boundaries, Hartmann (1991) cited case material suggesting that individuals with thick boundaries formed a strong identification with a parent of the same sex in childhood. These individuals also experienced markedly competitive feelings with older same-sex siblings and felt a need to grow up quickly. They developed a strong set of internalized rules and evidenced obsessive-compulsive traits. Hartmann (1991) found that individuals with thin boundaries failed to develop a strong identification with the same-sex parent, and experienced traumatic violations (e.g., sexual abuse). These findings are also consistent with studies suggesting a correlation between hypnotizability or proneness to fantasy and childhood trauma (Rhue and Lynn 1991).

Although Hartmann has developed an interesting and promising research tool that has opened a new window into the study of ego boundaries, the 145-item BQ in its present form seems unwieldy to administer and score. On the basis of its face content, it appears mainly to study "traits." Judging from Celenza's findings (1986) (she employed an earlier version of the BQ), the BQ does not assess the way an individual might respond to specific situations in which his or her external or internal boundaries are challenged in a stressful way.

The Holding Environment

To a greater or lesser degree, a patient temporarily suspends his or her critical judgment during treatment. In this state, the patient becomes in some ways like an infant who is unable to organize or process reality without the structuring influences of the parent's care. Winnicott (1960b/1965) conceptualized this scenario as the *holding environment*. In this situation, the mother is able to identify with her infant. She can perceive, in a "good enough" way, the infant's moment-to-moment needs for emotional regulation and physical care. Her response constitutes a real-time, "live adaptation" to the infant's requirements. The holding environment is like a construction scaffolding that supports the infant's developing ego boundaries.

In his observation of infants during the first 2 months of life, Spitz (1965) confirmed the idea of the *stimulus barrier* that provides them with a high threshold to external excitation. As the infant's threshold to stimuli diminishes, its rudimentary ego takes over the screening role of the barrier by processing internal and external stimuli. The primary caregiver (usually the mother) functions as an external ego boundary that augments the infant's internal stimulus barrier to excitation by providing emotional and physical regulation. Ordinary infant care, such as feeding, providing warmth, changing clothes, reducing noise, and soothing, can all be seen as stimulus reduction functions.

In Mahler's (1968) description of the subphases of separation-individuation, she emphasized that from 2 to 8 months of age, the infant is enclosed in a stimulus shield that represents a "highly selective boundary" containing the mother infant "dual unity." The mother functions as an "auxiliary ego," augmenting the infant's developing internal ego. During this period of dual unity, outside stimuli are dealt with by monitoring the mother's face and presence. This is a "biphasic" sensory processing in which everything is experienced with reference to the mother. Mahler likened the infant's emerging sense of interest in experiences occurring outside the dual unity to a "hatching" process. Differentiation takes place with the infant "checking back to the mother as a point of orientation" (see Figure 3–6).

Just as a parent's holding provides an initial regulatory environment in which an infant can begin to "hatch" and develop a progressive sense of "me-ness" with which to differentiate itself from the rest of the world, therapeutic holding provides a place in which a patient can begin to resolve conflicts and problems that center on trust and individuation. For very anxious and regressed patients, "checking in" with the therapist provides an immediate calming of emotional turmoil. Some patients report that just hearing the therapist's voice on their answering machine tape can calm them down during a crisis or anxiety attack. If certain patients sense that the therapist is uninterested, unenthusiastic, or cold, they are likely to reject the treatment and drop out prematurely. On the other hand, a distorted or seductive form of "holding" geared to the therapist's needs rather than to the specific moment-to-moment needs of the patient interferes with the treatment process and is likely to compound the patient's psychopathology.

The psychotherapy frame recapitulates the boundary-defining function of the child's early holding environment. All psychotherapy patients have a regressive component to their problems that may manifest in the treatment relationship. Whether or not the therapist encourages overt exploration of these dependent longings, the therapist should be aware of them and have an organized and coherent framework with which to contain them. The psychotherapist's ability to regulate the therapeutic environment is analogous to the parental "holding" function. By keeping boundaries, the therapist configures a framework within which the patient can be safe yet spontaneous. The treatment boundaries need to be of optimal permeability, in the sense that they are neither too thick nor too thin. At the same time, they must adapt dynamically to the patient's needs of the moment.

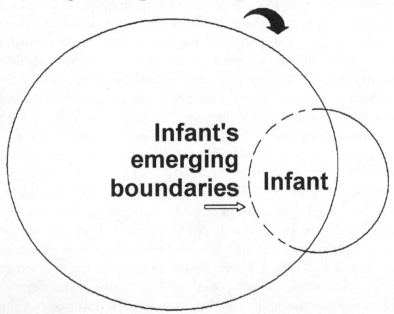

Figure 3–6. The parent's ego boundaries function as a holding environment for the infant during its "hatching" process. The infant's boundaries are highly permeable (*dotted portion of circle*). Its thinking is characterized predominantly by primary process. As the infant "hatches" from the protective enclosure provided by the parent's ego boundaries, it gradually develops its own ability to employ secondary process (*solid portion of circle*) and to "classify" the world.

The "holding" function in infancy refers to emotional holding and physical care. In psychotherapy with outpatients, holding is symbolically represented by the presence, warmth, patience, understanding, and responsiveness of the therapist as well as by his or her familiar, secure physical setting. *Holding* does not imply literal hugging, embrace, or any form of pleasure-giving physical touch, although it is construed in this way by some therapists. Patients may experience medication as a form of holding in that it functions as an actual physical substance given by the therapist to relieve symptoms and regulate distress. With acutely suicidal patients, therapeutic "holding" may necessitate physically taking hold of the patient if he or she needs to be brought to the hospital for safety.

In its most concrete application, therapeutic holding involves being able to contain the patient's psychopathology for the patient's benefit. Patients respond positively, on both conscious and unconscious levels, to a therapist who provides a stable holding environment. On a primary process level, they experience a sense of relative trust, confidence, hope, and safety. These are visceral, "coenesthetic" responses. On a more rational and logical level, the same therapist will inspire thoughts such as "he or she is organized, intelligent, capable, friendly, sympathetic, and understanding."

The Psychotherapist and the Legal Concept of the "Common Carrier"

The "holding" metaphor emphasizes how vulnerable our patients can feel when they entrust themselves to our care. This metaphor can also help us to understand the symbolic elaborations of patients' unconscious feelings about psychotherapy. The symbolic experience of being held is verified by the fact that many patients report imagery linking the treatment process to a vehicular conveyance. They often dream about their therapy in terms of a trip taken by car, bus, train, plane, or boat. This image is an interesting one because it combines the idea of being carried with the wish to be taken on a gratifying journey.

From this point of view, the psychotherapist and his or her treatment frame can be likened to a *common carrier*, as the term is employed in the law. A common carrier is a company that transports passengers and goods from place to place. The law requires that such companies pursue the "utmost care" and the "vigilance of a very cautious person" in serving the passengers who have consigned their persons into the conveyance (*Cooper v. National Railroad Passenger Corp. et al.* 1975). In the same way, a psychotherapy patient has paid a fee and entrusted mind and body to a process that contains and carries (Bion 1970/1977). Some patients are as vulnerable as a baby in its parent's arms. Such patients are prime targets for therapeutic exploitation.

The concept of psychotherapy as a vehicle of transport that "contains" the patient was suggested by Freud's way of explaining the use of free association to new analytic patients:

> Act as though, for instance, you were a traveler sitting next to the window of a railway carriage and describing to someone inside the carriage the changing views which you see outside. (Freud 1913/1958, p. 135)

A clinical example of the therapeutic frame as a vehicle can be seen in the following dream of a psychotherapy patient during the final weeks of terminating his treatment. He had frequently dreamed about the therapy in terms of buses and trains:

> I watched the analyst walking into her house. I was saying good-bye. I saw she had a catamaran, a twin-hulled vessel, in the garage. I was thinking, "So you have a boat, also?"

On its surface level, the dream as analyzed from the patient's associations recapitulated oral, anal, phallic, and oedipal issues connected with the patient's attachment to the therapist. Also present were both feelings of longing for sexual conquest and fears of castration. At a more basic level, however, the dream portrayed the patient's feeling that his therapist had kept him afloat for many years during the treatment. The twin-hulled vessel was equivalent to her body that was unified and linked in a twinship with his own. The termination issue that he had to resolve involved his wish to travel along in his *own* independent vessel. He had finally begun to experience his body as intact and separate from hers.

One of Winnicott's (1963/1965) patients also employed a transportational metaphor to portray her experience of therapy as she struggled with strong dependency conflicts during the early phases of psychoanalysis. She reacted to the analyst's separation as a form of annihilation. She dreamed of herself as a horse that "had to be shot, else it would have kicked its way out of an airplane."

Transitional Objects, the "False Self," and Role Reversal

Anything that interferes with the parent's role in providing an auxiliary ego boundary tends to force the infant to rely prematurely on its own inadequate resources. Such a crisis leads to pathological thickening of the ego boundaries at a stage of development when those boundaries should be highly porous. Mahler (1968) saw this as a factor in the later development of an "as if" personality. Winnicott (1960b/1965) described the same phenomenon in terms of the infant's forming a *false self*. Although in some aspects the false self represents our social "face" in nonintimate relations, in its pathological manifestations it develops from a compliant adaptation to a parent who is unable to accept and contain the infant's spontaneous gestures and playful creations. Winnicott (1960c/1965) considered this adaptation to be a result of the parent's inability to form a holding environment in which the infant could take joy in its illusory "transitional" experiences. He employed the term *transitional* (Winnicott 1951/1958) to describe the way that infants 4–12 months old tried to adapt to environmental changes. For example, a blanket or a wisp of hair can become charged with emotional feeling and serve as a comforting substitute for the mother while the baby is going to sleep. The infant's ability to use the blanket to create an illusion that is itself soothing takes place within the safety of the holding environment. In this way, the infant forms a sense of being a unique self that acquires an *internal* ability to modulate emotions.

Premature renunciation of these illusions may lead to serious character problems and psychopathology, such as alexithymia or the "as if" personality (Krystal 1988; Mahler 1968; Winnicott 1960b/ 1965). A similar phenomenon occurs if the parent becomes overly anxious or rejecting as a result of the child's increasing efforts at individuation and mobility during the "practicing" period from 9 to 18 months of age (Mahler 1968). Although on the surface the child may appear compliant, internally he or she must suppress awareness of the burgeoning desire to be a separate and unique individual. In the most severe cases, the child may have difficulty learning to use symbols for communication or expressing feelings. He or she may come to associate efforts at competent achievement with an inner sense of shame and personal defectiveness (Nathanson 1992). Greenspan's (1992a) videotaped recordings of mother-infant interactions poignantly demonstrated this process:

> A mother held a squeeze toy in front of her 8-month-old baby. Although the baby appeared interested at first, the mother continued to squeak the squeeze toy in a perseverative rhythm as if to the tune of a different drummer, without synchrony with, or awareness of the baby's efforts to touch it or develop an interest in it. After several attempts to interact with the toy, during which the mother squeaked it at him instead of letting him explore it himself at his own pace, the baby plopped over like a limp doll and began to cough.

Here is another example of this phenomenon drawn from an observation of a toddler:

> Sally was 15 months old when her mother became depressed. Prior to her mother's depression, Sally and she had interacted in a natural and cheerful way. Since the onset of her mood disturbance, mother had become somewhat dependent on Sally's smile to cheer her up. I evaluated Sally in a session when she was 18 months of age. Her play was very low key and methodical, without much joy. When Sally saw that I had a glass of water on a table from which I had taken a drink during the play, she looked at the glass. She then looked back at me and grunted. She placed a toy in front of me, looked at the glass of water again, grunted, looked back at me and

gave me another toy. She repeated this process about three or four times, until there was a pile of toys in front of me. She was showering me with tribute. I realized at that point that she was "paying" me to give her a drink of water.

Sally's behavior was an example of premature development. She had to "compensate" me for gratification, just as she had to cheer up her mother to receive care. This is an example of role reversal in a caregiving situation. The child felt impelled to act in a parental role and to gratify the adult. In role reversal, the caregiver needs or expects the baby to be "entertaining," to "be good," or to be comforting, without sufficient sense of the baby's own needs. To the extent that a child is deprived of the parent's "holding" boundary, that child is forced to rely prematurely on his or her own devices. In its most extreme form, a child's need to comply is seen in the bland expressionlessness and accommodation of abused children (Summit 1983). This precocious assumption of what might later be seen as a normal social role (i.e., being thoughtful about another person's needs) can be pathological because the child is pushed into taking on this burden at a time when he or she is cognitively and emotionally unprepared to do so. As a result, the internalized ego state that represents "the self that takes care of others" may be conceptualized as possessing an unnaturally thick boundary and will be relatively disconnected from the rest of the personality (see Figure 3–2). This is why such ego states are often perceived to be "false" in the way Winnicott (1960b/1965) used the term.

Traumatic experiences that are combined with inappropriate role reversal during childhood are frequently reported by patients seeking psychotherapy. Clinical observation shows that role reversal is often observed in individuals raised by alcoholic, depressed, psychotic, or abusive parents. Role reversal in childhood can be particularly confusing when combined with excessive gratification and seduction. Examples include parental overindulgence, incest, and overly intense investment in a particular quality of a child that satisfies a parent's own needs. Inappropriate role reversal interferes with the child's ability to use the transitional experiences that are needed to form a coherent sense of self.

Tabin (1992) has theorized that transitional objects protect against narcissistic injury in later stages of development. As an illustration, Tabin (1992) described the way a teenager might use a transitional object such as a small stuffed animal to cope with an incompletely organized aspect of the self. Transitional objects are thought to strengthen ego boundaries and to protect adolescents against emotions, such as shame and anger, that could threaten their sense of self-integration. A stuffed animal can be imbued with the qualities that the teenager desires to possess in a more permanent way. As a proxy of the self, it provides a method of maintaining inner mastery and control. For adults, a familiar object such as a wallet photograph helps to maintain a reminder of home while away on a trip. Like a nomad's tent, it can be used as a portable enclosure that retains an element of constancy in the midst of an ever-changing landscape.

Within the holding structure of the adequately defined treatment frame, the patient is safe to communicate his or her distress, conflicts, fantasies, and projections. The therapeutic boundaries define a space within which the patient may play and experiment with those perceptions that lie in a twilight zone between fantasy and reality. The therapist must be careful to respect the "transitional" nature of these communications. They are the patient's creations, similar to the transitional phenomena experienced by infants.

Patients learn better how to deal with frightening internal states if the therapist is able to convey through word and gesture that he or she can be related to in a symbolic rather than literal way. Even if a patient's mental productions consist of sexual overtures, sadistic fantasies, or persecutory delusions, as long as they are kept within the confines of the treatment boundaries, the therapist should remember to respect their symbolic nature. The patient may attempt to break the therapeutic framework by acting out these illusions in a potentially harmful way. In such a case, the therapist must be careful to focus initial interventions at the level of the boundary rather than on the content of the fantasy.

For example, if a therapist starts taking a patient's sexual fantasies literally by responding in kind instead of treating them as a "transitional" process to be "contained," the patient is likely to become confused and disoriented, because the illusory "playacting" aspect of his or her communication has been disrupted. As another illustration, if a patient has acted on a sadistic fantasy with a third person, he or she can misinterpret a tone of annoyance or criticism in the therapist's response as a rejection of the fantasy rather than as a concern about safety. As a way of guarding against this confusion, the therapist might appropriately say:

> It is important that we understand the basis of your desires, but we are less likely to be able to find out why this is so important to you if you continue to put it into action instead of talking about it with me.

The treatment boundaries, the psychotherapist, and other members of a treatment team such as nursing staff may be employed in this way as transitional objects (Epstein 1982). The therapist's office itself and its contents may also become invested as transitional objects. For example, many patients become attached to items in the office such as paintings, a particular piece of furniture, a pillow, bric-a-brac, or a tissue box. The therapist's voice on the answering machine and the familiar voices of the answering service operators can function in the same way. The therapist's guidelines become familiar landmarks that enable the patient to develop his or her own ability to contain distressing affects. By employing these seemingly trivial yet very comforting aspects of the therapy setting in their own idiosyncratic and personally creative ways, patients can experience them as a part of themselves—a soothing possession internalized as a part of their own permanent psychic structure. The therapeutic boundaries comprise the physical setting, the regularity of the visits, the person of the therapist, and the reliable guidelines. These boundaries form a therapeutic space in which the patient is free both to be creative and to heal injuries in his or her sense of self. As Viderman (1974) pointed out, serious deviations in the boundaries constrict the space and prevent spontaneous expression of certain conflicts and issues. The therapist's personality plays an important role in shaping the treatment boundaries so that they are neither too thick nor too thin. According to Kohut (quoted by Freinhar 1986):

> The good analyst will have a personality that is characterized by "central firmness and peripheral looseness . . . changeableness, and impressionability," which will allow [him or her] to respond with respect and empathic comprehension to all [the] patient's productions. (Freinhar 1986, p. 483)

Therapists with overly thick boundaries are likely to prematurely close off the patient's spontaneous expression. Such therapists are less sensitive to the patient's efforts to communicate through primary process symbolization. They employ excessive advice and are prone to rush their patients into relinquishing symptoms before they are ready. Under the care of a thick-boundaried therapist, a patient who employs a significant "false self" defense might appear to improve behaviorally as part of that accommodative style. However, the patient's problems may later manifest in ways that are less amenable to treatment.

Therapists with overly thin boundaries are likely to confuse their intrapsychic experience of the patient with the actual patient. These therapists have difficulty differentiating the patient's space from their own, tend to be excessively friendly and familiar, and are more likely to use touch. Although they may be very attuned to the patient's feelings and symbolic communications, they have a problem applying this information in its proper context. For example, if a patient is angry, a therapist with excessively thin boundaries might find it impossible to keep that emotion distinct from his or her own feelings and behavior. Thin-boundaried therapists tend to infantilize their patients and to promote unnecessary regression. Although a patient may improve symptomatically for a while, he or she is deprived of the opportunity to learn new ways of adapting to environmental and interpersonal stresses.

Therapists may simultaneously possess excessively thick boundaries in some respects and overly thin boundaries in others. For example, a therapist may treat a patient as an extension of his or her own body and become involved in a sexual relationship (excessive thinness) at the same time that he or she expects the patient to relinquish all symptoms and become the new therapist in a reversal of roles (excessive thickness).

The Effect of Pathological
Narcissism on Ego Boundaries

Pathological narcissism is like the "dry rot" of ego boundaries. It may not look that serious in an otherwise well-functioning person, but when stressed, the surface caves in. Individuals suffering from narcissistic pathology are impaired in their ability to regulate feelings of shame (Nathanson 1992; O'Leary and Wright 1986). As a result, therapists afflicted with such problems are seriously hampered in their ability to stay focused on patients' needs without confusing them with their own (Finell 1985; O'Leary and Wright 1986; Welt and Herron 1990; Wurmser 1987). Self-deception and a sense of "specialness" provide a fertile growth medium for abuse of power and the exploitation of patients (Epstein and Simon 1990). A review of narcissistic development is therefore quite relevant to the issue of boundary maintenance.

In Kohut's (1971) view, a child's healthy narcissism develops as a result of his or her dealing with gradual frustrations in a supportive and empathic environment. The child's grandiose aspirations for inner perfection (the *grandiose self*) and, later on, his or her need to be united in loving relation with an idealized caregiver (the *idealized selfobject*) are stages in forming a coherent "self." Kohut's use of the term *self* can be construed as being equivalent to either a single internalized ego state or a person's entire system of ego states. The child gradually internalizes the caregivers' empathic "holding" as a permanent part of his or her psychic structure (Tolpin 1972). A coherent treatment frame functions in the same way.

According to Kohut (1971), pathologic narcissism develops because the child's caregivers are unable to provide adequate empathic holding. In contrast to Kohut's developmental deficit theory, Kernberg (1975) focused more on intrapsychic conflict to explain narcissistic pathology (Glassman 1988). Both Kohut (1971) and Kernberg (1975) observed that the parents of narcissistic patients have an impaired ability to relate to their children's own dependency needs. At the same time, the parents become overinvested in gratifying themselves with the child's "special" giftedness or attractiveness.

Used and perceived as part-objects by their parents, these children learn to perceive themselves and others as objects to be exploited rather than to be related to as whole individuals. As for the "special" gifts, whether they reflected good looks, wealth, intellectual brilliance, or musical talent, these qualities become experienced as brittle and desperate substitutes for genuine relatedness. They evolve as the organizing foci of the pathological frame that the patient brings into psychotherapy. A positive attribute that is discerned as a "booby prize" becomes a meager compensation for an inner feeling of hollowness and low self-esteem. It is the foundation for a "false self."

Kohut (1971) observed that individuals with a grandiose type of narcissism suffered from a "vertical split" in their psyches consisting of a shame-filled, low-esteem "reality ego" on the one hand, and a disavowed but openly "exhibitionistic self" on the other. This grandiose and exhibitionistic self is derived from the parents' exploitation of the child's performance. It represents the way the person was "spoiled" and seduced with a "booby prize."

It is possible to conceptualize pathological narcissism as related to deformations in the therapist's ego boundaries, and therefore to his or her treatment boundaries. I have developed a model that I have found clinically useful in understanding the boundary problems experienced by narcissistic therapists. Derived primarily from the work of J. G. and H. H. Watkins (1982, 1990, 1993) and of Kohut (1971), it attempts to explain the confusing mixture of "looseness" and defensive rigidity manifest in narcissistic therapists in terms of distortions in the configuration of their internal and external boundaries. A therapist burdened with significant narcissistic pathology will tend to relate to a patient as if he or she were an idealized internal possession (selfobject) rather than an independent person. Although this situation may promote a certain degree of empathy, more likely than not it will also interfere with the therapist's ability to understand and adapt to the patient's real problems. For example, some therapists place excessive reliance on the feelings of gratification they obtain from their patients' appealing qualities, such as sexual attractiveness, intelligence, wealth, or worldly accomplishments. These clinicians have a greater tendency to turn a blind eye to any information that would cast the patient in a bad light because they experience such data as a painful disillusionment that deflates the value of an ideal-ized possession. Although relatively healthy in most other aspects of life, their external boundaries become overly permeable when they come into close contact with patients whose special qualities resonate with their defensive needs. Narcissistic therapists also evidence what may be termed a defensively overvalued ego state. This is manifested clinically by a grandiose attitude that is relatively impervious to logi-cal arguments or educative efforts, because it serves as a rigid defense against warded-off feelings of internalized shame (see Figure 3–7).

Shame as a "Regulator" of Ego Boundaries and Social Interaction

Shame has been described as one of the primary human affects (Nathanson 1992). It appears to modulate interpersonal relationships and social bonding. It has been my observation that maladaptive defenses against feelings of shame play a critical role in therapeutic boundary violations. For this reason, I believe it would be useful to review some of the literature on this subject. A more detailed discus-sion of shame mechanisms in boundary violations is presented in subsequent chapters.

Tomkins (1987) considered shame as a regulatory affect that serves to inhibit the emotions of interest and enjoyment. Shame is usually an intensely disruptive feeling. It is the emotion experienced when a person's relational frame has been broken. In contrast, feel-ings of guilt are organized around actual or fantasied behavior. The basic internal message associated with guilt is "My actions are the problem." With shame, the individual's global sense of self-worth is diminished. Its basic internal message is "I am the problem."

Lansky (1992) clarified some of the different semantic uses of the term *shame*. Individuals who employ *signal* shame are alerted to the fact that a social bond is being threatened. This allows them to at-tempt adaptive means to repair the breach. The term may also be applied to the devastating feelings that are experienced if a social connection has been ruptured, as well as to the pathological reactions that follow. In the active sense of the term, "to shame" another

Narcissistic therapist's
ego boundaries

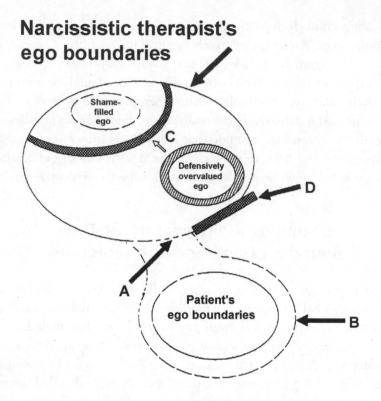

Figure 3–7. Hypothesized model explaining the mechanism by which pathological narcissism interferes with a therapist's ability to maintain treatment boundaries. Therapists with a significant degree of pathological narcissism appear to have porous defects in segments of their boundaries (A). In certain interpersonal contexts, they are impaired in their ability to separate fantasy from reality and "me" from "not-me." Such therapists tend to overidentify with the special qualities in their patients and to perceive them as if they were an idealized part of themselves. The therapist's fantasized experience of the patient as a part of himself or herself is portrayed in the diagram as an outpouching of the therapist's external ego boundary (B), such that the patient is perceived as if he or she were one of the therapist's internalized ego states. This narcissistic idealization of the patient assists the therapist in warding off the awareness of his or her own feelings of shame. In addition, the defensively overvalued ego state operating within the therapist forms a relatively impermeable defense against feelings of shame by sustaining a barrier against internalized shame states (C) and by promoting a pathological "thickening" in the external boundary (D). This barrier tends to block out realistic but potentially disappointing information about the "real" as opposed to the "narcissistically perceived" patient.

person can be seen either as a well-intentioned effort to administer corrective discipline or as a hostile way of wreaking psychological destruction. C. D. Schneider (1987) emphasized that in its most mature form, a "sense of shame" is consistent with the civilized way that people show concern and sensitivity to one another. "Mature" shame is reflected in tactfulness, modesty, a sense of awe, and a respect for both one's own and another's need for privacy.

Nathanson (1987, 1992) interpreted Spitz's (1965) observations of 6- to 8-month-old infants during the phase of "stranger anxiety" as one of the earliest manifestations of shame. Babies at this age will no longer smile indiscriminately when presented with a human face. Only a familiar person will stimulate that special sense of excitement and delight. Upon seeing a stranger, a baby will lower its eyes, appear shy, cover its face, close its eyes, hide behind something, throw itself down, weep, or scream (Spitz 1965). Broucek (1982) pointed out that infants at this stage will also manifest archaic feelings of shame on occasions when the mother herself is perceived as a stranger—for instance, if she is in a bad mood, or tired, or ill. Seen in this context, shame is the affect that accompanies any interruption in excitement, interest, or involvement with familiar caregivers. As such, it operates as a social organizer and is thus intimately connected with the formation of self-image and ego boundaries.

Because shame is an important social modifier in the formation of boundaries and social mores, it plays an important role in modifying an individual's comprehension of what is happening in an interpersonal relationship. Shame is disruptive to an individual's ability to learn and participate in interactions with others. When shame is too intense, it can lead to impaired cognition. Nathanson (1987) postulated that the facial flushing and erythema commonly associated with the experience of shame may be connected with a corresponding cerebral vasodilation that impairs cognition.

Experimental work suggests that an individual's level of perceived shame appears to correlate with certain measurable psychological characteristics. Lewis (1971, 1987) reviewed studies of the relationship between shame and *field independence*. When placed in a darkened room, field-independent individuals are able to distinguish when an illuminated rod superimposed over an illuminated frame is truly vertical, regardless of whether the frame has been tilted at an angle. Field-independent subjects are also better able to distinguish a simple object that is embedded in a complex pictorial design. Conversely, *field dependent* individuals are less able to distinguish between foreground and background. Parkes (1982) noted that field-dependent subjects are more global and less perceptually discriminating than are field-independent subjects. As a result, field-dependent individuals tend to blur the boundaries between conceptual categories with regard to their inner experiences and psychological perceptions. Other studies have shown that field-dependent individuals are more prone to express feelings of shame in psychotherapy (Lewis 1971, 1987).

In her review of the literature on the subject, Lewis (1971) remarked that field-dependent individuals were more likely to have a global, relatively unarticulated concept of the human body; to come from an environment that emphasized obedience rather than initiative and independence; and to score high on tests of suggestibility. These findings suggest that field-dependent patients might be more likely to confuse transference with reality. Such individuals also are likely to be more vulnerable to exploitation by therapists because of their cognitive problems in distinguishing between the therapeutic "frame" and the "content" of the treatment. Although less experimental evidence exists regarding field-dependent psychotherapists (Lewis 1971), it is reasonable to expect that they, too, are more prone to have difficulty with feelings of shame, and to have problems in maintaining a therapeutic frame in the face of treatment events that threaten their sense of self-esteem.

In its more primitive and destructive forms, shame can be an extremely disruptive emotion. It is often associated with the feeling that one's self is splitting into pieces, as well as with an intense desire to hide or break off contact with others. As a result, intense shame is rarely allowed to stay in its free and undefended form for very long. Various defenses are deployed to cover it over, such as escape from social involvement, denial, dissociation, substance abuse, compulsive sex, compulsive self-deprecation, self-destructive behavior, grandiose feelings of entitlement, manic triumph, compulsive exhibitionism, haughtiness, sarcasm, teasing, jokes that ridicule, rage, and vengeful retaliation. Nathanson (1992) theorized that these defenses could be organized along two axes that he called "The Compass of Shame" (p. 312). Although presented as a way of identifying each individual's predominant defense against shame, his descriptive schema can be seen as a two-dimensional circumplex defining various mixtures of defenses. The first dimension is determined by an individual's proclivity for internalization versus externalization, characterized by the "attack other" defense at one pole and the "attack self" defense at the other. The second dimension reflects a person's temporal ability to sustain and experience shame affects, and consists of the shameful "withdrawal" defense at one pole and the narcissistic "avoidance" defense at the other. Nathanson (1992) defined *withdrawal* as an immediate way of escaping, *along with one's perceived feelings of shame*, to a location that is removed from the watchful presence of other persons who might be scornful or rejecting. *Avoidance* employs a more prolonged and compulsive use of behavioral and psychological devices to *obliterate* feelings of shame, such as the use of dissociation, addictive substances, overeating, hypersexuality, excessive risk taking, pressured overactivity, or hypomanic denial. In the conceptual model I have diagrammed in Figure 3–7, the internal and external arrangements used by the narcissistic therapist to prevent the experience of shame illustrate the mechanism of the "avoidance" defense. In subsequent chapters, I refer to all four of these basic defenses in analyzing some of the ways that therapists become involved in boundary violations.

Lazare (1992) emphasized how easy it is for therapists to overlook their patients' feelings of humiliation. Morrison (1983) stressed that it was important for therapists to acknowledge and understand their own painful shame affects in connection with any sense of internal deficiency or failure to reach life goals. The patient's shame may be stirred up as a result of having been "labeled" with a specific mental disorder, by the process of psychotherapy itself, and/or by specific attitudes of or comments by the therapist that the patient perceives as mortifying.

Lewis (1987) reported a vignette from a psychotherapy session that illustrated the way that patients experience shame when therapy boundaries are violated:

A therapist failed to keep a session. He had been unable to notify
the patient about it, and she had come for her appointment when
he wasn't there. At the next session, the therapist failed to recognize the patient's unconscious references to the feelings of shame
she experienced as a result of her sensing that she wasn't very
important to him. By the end of the session, the patient was blaming *herself* for having a problem of forgetting appointments. Instead
of taking responsibility for his own lapse and the effect it had on
the patient, the therapist agreed with her self-effacing comments.

Analyzing this case in terms of Nathanson's (1992) descriptive
schema, the therapist defended against his shame primarily by using
the "attack other" mode, whereas the patient relied mainly upon an
"attack self" strategy.

Therapists who have difficulty dealing appropriately with feelings
of shame also have trouble establishing reliable boundaries with their
patients. Problems may arise either because they are inattentive to
this issue or because they fear they will devastate the patient if they
bring up the subject of shame. For example, in a situation where a
patient makes a direct sexual overture, the therapist might haughtily
inform the patient:

Our relationship is not going to be a sexual one.

Because this statement is made in a smug and arrogant way without
being accompanied by an empathic effort to understand how spurned
and hurt the patient might feel, the therapist is denying his or her
own sense of vulnerability and is unwittingly shaming the patient.
The therapist is defending against a perceived weakness in his or her
own ego boundaries by projecting it onto the patient. This therapist's
defensive tactics would appear to involve both "avoidance" (grandiose disavowal) and a subtle measure of "attack other." As a result, the
therapist has lost touch with the patient's sense of exposure. Alternatively, if the therapist responds to the patient's sexual overture by
blushing and saying

Oh, I feel the same way about you, but I'm worried my spouse
might get suspicious if we got involved in an affair.

this therapist would be defending against feelings of shame by using a combination of "withdrawal" and "attack self" strategies. On a conscious level, such a clinician might seem anxious, at any cost, to protect the patient from feeling the humiliation of rejection. Unfortunately, such a response would sabotage the opportunity to help the patient learn a more adaptive way of dealing with shame and is likely to be confusing as well, because the boundary was linked to the social convention of adultery, rather than to the therapist's desire to safeguard the patient and his or her treatment.

Projective Identification and Introjective Identification as Modes of Communication During Conditions of High Boundary Permeability

The mode of communication between two persons is closely related to the permeability of their ego boundaries. Interactions in which one or both participants have very porous boundaries can give rise to projective identification and introjective identification. These are special ways of conveying information that are highly imbued with primary process thinking. It is important that therapists be able to recognize and work with these mechanisms as part of the treatment process, because many patients will regress to a more primitive form of interaction during treatment. Such regression can occur either as a consequence of serious psychopathology or as a derivative of the nonverbal component of distressing memories. Monitoring projective identification and introjective identification during treatment often assists therapists in achieving a deeper understanding of their patients' problems. By selectively increasing the permeability of their ego boundaries, therapists are able to be more receptive to their patients' communications.

The term *projective identification* was originally employed by Melanie Klein (1946) to describe the way that infants rid themselves of unbearable mental contents by externalizing them onto their primary caregivers. For example, when a hungry baby cries in rage and anguish, the mother experiences its distress and feels emotionally impelled to respond. Klein (1946, p. 102) postulated that the infant experiences its rage as a fantasy to "suck dry, bite up, scoop out and rob the mother's body of its good contents" and to expel "dangerous substances (excrement) out of the self and into the mother." According to Klein (1946), the infant experiences these aggressive impulses as a threat to its coherence: "under the pressure of this threat the ego tends to fall to bits" (p. 101). A defensive maneuver she called *splitting* is employed to separate the "good" (fulfilling) mother/breast from the "bad" (frustrating) one. Splitting results in a "dispersal of the destructive impulse which is felt as the source of danger" (p. 101). Projective identification refers to this process of extruding the "bad" parts of the self, which are then reingested as an introject. *Reingestion* refers to the process of "introjective identification," in which externalized qualities are taken into the system. The infant's developing sense of control is closely tied to this reingestion of evacuated contents.

The infant's perceptual universe may be compared to a chamber of mirrors, in which any mental activity or emotion can be destructively (or constructively) reflected back upon its source in an infinite series of projective and introjective identifications. To use a thermodynamic analogy, what starts out as a simple system with two degrees of freedom (i.e., inside me *or* inside you) multiplies exponentially to infinite complexity (i.e., what was inside me is now in you, but is then taken again inside me . . . etc.).

Although Winnicott (1962/1965) felt that Klein's concepts were clinically useful, he argued that they did not sufficiently emphasize the importance of the mother's role in the equation, and he cautioned against ascribing such differentiated imagery to infants in the first 8 months of life.

Kernberg (1975) used the concept of projective identification to explain the intense and unstable transference-countertransference phenomena in the treatment of borderline patients. For example, a patient may deal with his vituperative rage by projecting it onto the therapist. Instead of fearing his own destructive self-criticism, the patient now believes that the therapist hates him and is viciously demeaning of him, and will feel impelled to control the therapist by various means such as appeasement, flight, manipulation, or counter-attack. The patient's accusations and manipulative behavior are likely to stimulate anger and critical feelings in the therapist. Even though the patient may retain strong ego boundaries in other areas of his life, a blurring of the distinction between himself and the therapist will tend to facilitate projective identification, and will in turn be intensified by the ensuing enmeshment. This outcome is particularly likely to occur if the therapist becomes worn down by the stress of the patient's manipulativeness and acts out the projected affects, thereby confirming their reality in the patient's mind. It is for this reason that Kernberg (1975) emphasized the importance of firm adherence to therapeutic boundaries in treating borderline patients.

The use of projective identification involves a mental splitting of the caregiving parent into "all good" or "all bad" parts. Splitting results from the unbearable tension produced by the need for the regulatory soothing of a "good" (i.e., gratifying) parent who is sometimes experienced as "bad" (i.e., nongratifying or rejecting). From work with older children and adults, one can infer that projective identification is experienced at a visceral level that evokes internal imagery such as spitting, screaming, defecation, and vomiting. This sense of throwing out the "bad" contents onto the mother portrays the infant as attempting to process and detoxify its unbearable psychic tension by evacuation. It is a primitive, global, gestural, and *coenesthetically* organized form of interacting.

As a mechanism that originally takes place at a developmental stage at which the distinction between self and other is quite blurred, the identification phase of projective identification follows from the sense that "outside" is not much different than "inside." The idea of the talion dread (i.e., that one will be punished according to the principle of "an eye for an eye and a tooth for a tooth") stems from this blurring of inside and outside and forms an important part of the mental imagery and vengefulness in projective identification.

Although I have emphasized their heavy reliance on primary process thinking, projective identification and introjective identification are not always negative or pathological. Within certain constraints, these mechanisms are responsible for much of the "poetry" and "sweet mystery" of human relationships. Projective and introjective identification form the unconscious substrate for a large portion of the bonding and interaction that take place within romantic relationships, family ties, close friendships, group cohesion, and the patient-therapist dyad. In studying the nature of projective identification in family systems that contain adolescents, Zinner and Shapiro (1972) concluded that whereas all families employ these mechanisms, the negative or positive consequences depend on the contextual meaning of the projections and introjections exchanged between parent and child.

As a clinical concept, projective identification is extremely useful to therapists as a way of attending to a patient's emotional state. By observing their own tensions, anxiety, anger, hatred, guilt, boredom, submissiveness, and erotic desires, therapists are in a position to *infer* the existence of corresponding mental states operating in their patients that are being projected outward. In his classic paper on countertransference, Racker (1957) described this same phenomenon (without using the term *projective identification*) as the "complementary countertransference." If a patient is angry and critical of the therapist, the therapist starts to feel like a guilty and submissive child. Racker described how every positive transference is answered by a positive countertransference in the therapist, while every negative transference is answered by a negative countertransference. On an unconscious level, the therapist may be tempted to answer a negative transference (e.g., the patient is critical) with a talion response such as ending the session early. For this reason, it is essential that the therapist analyze his or her own emotional responses to avoid acting out these feelings.

Roland (1981) argued that not all emotional reactions that therapists experience in the therapy setting should be considered countertransference in the classical sense of an unconscious or neurotic reaction to the patient's transference. Rather, some may be precipitated by the patient's unconscious schemata—in other words, a script is being reenacted in which the therapist is assigned a role, like a character in a play.

Some therapists tend to take these projected feelings literally, as if the strange and alien emotions and fantasies evoked in them by a patient automatically provided a one-to-one correlation with the patient's experiences. Finell (1986) cautioned against relying on projective identification as a magical and semi-omnipotent technique for reading the patient's mind. Even if the therapist registers the projected emotion accurately, the patient's conflicts and the ways the therapist processes and reacts to them are rarely in perfect synchrony. A danger exists that the therapist will become intoxicated by the diffusion of ego boundaries and experience this state as a mystical union. It is important for each therapist to look at his or her own idiosyncratic reactions to the patient's issues.

Racker (1957) reasoned that in most circumstances, it is preferable for the therapist to begin by exploring his or her own countertransference feelings, and then to attempt to find out what the patient is thinking or feeling about the therapist's state of mind. For example, the therapist might inquire, "Are you aware of any thoughts or fantasies of how I might be feeling about you right now?" In this way the patient is given the opportunity to experience ownership of the projected emotions, based on his or her own thoughts or feelings, rather than to have them presented by the therapist as a magically experienced "reading of minds." Similarly, Roland (1981) argued that the patient may feel burdened if the therapist reveals his or her own feelings based on projective identification. Although the patient might be very impressed by the therapist's ability to "know" what he or she is feeling, making such a revelation risks encouraging further projective identification by increasing the blur in the boundaries between them. Helping the patient to discover the projected part on his or her own will strengthen boundaries.

Most of the confusion about the concept of projective identification centers around distinguishing it from projection proper, and the idea of whether the projected contents represent a self or an object representation. W. N. Goldstein (1991) has provided a thorough and excellent review in this regard.

As previously mentioned, the twin concepts of introjective and projective identification refer to the ability of one person to internalize a complex mental representation projected by another. The internalized contents need not be considered an "introject" in the classical psychoanalytic sense of *an internally perceived part of the self*. As both Schafer (1968) and Roland (1981) have pointed out, the internalized material may be considered "primary process presences" consisting not only of introjects but also of conscious or unconscious scripts, attitudes, and ways of viewing oneself, one's primary caregivers, and the world. In this sense, these "presences" can be seen as the basic units for the social frames that Goffman (1974) described.

In the therapy setting, if the introjected contents are successfully "metabolized," they can be handed back in a modified and "detoxified" form. The therapist can "reframe" a negative experience so that it seems less upsetting:

> Dr. Baldwin felt anxious when Mr. Culp began to criticize her in the following way: "You don't give me the advice I need, you don't encourage me enough, and you're just not helping me!"
>
> Dr. Baldwin started to feel very unworthy and ineffectual, despite the fact that Mr. Culp seemed to have been making considerable progress during the 8 months he had been in therapy. She was able to connect her own emotions to Mr. Culp's early memories of being criticized by his obsessional mother. She calmly said to him: "I can tell that you're very upset with me today and I'd like to understand it better. I'm a little puzzled because the other day you seemed to be telling me how things were going better. Tell me, does what's happening between us here today remind you of anything that's happened to you before?"
>
> Mr. Culp thought about this for a while and replied: "Yes. My mother used to yell at me about all sorts of shortcomings. She would always compare me to my cousins or the neighbor's kids. They were supposedly smarter, neater, or better behaved than I was. I tried so hard to please her. Just when I thought I had done something good so she'd give me a smile, she'd find something else wrong."
>
> Dr. Baldwin responded: "It had to be pretty demoralizing for you. No matter what you did, you found she was unhappy about it. Could that be something like the way it's working in here between you and me today? You seemed to be finding a lot of fault with me a few minutes ago."
>
> Mr. Culp laughed: "Now you know what it was like for me!"

In this example, Dr. Baldwin was able to maintain a strong treatment boundary that "contained" the patient's projections. She was able to listen to and contain her fears of being ineffectual. In so doing, she was able to understand her patient better. Rather than becoming argumentative or countercritical, she was able to talk to him about what *he* might be experiencing, in a calm and caring way. In this situation, the patient was given an opportunity to reintroject the formerly "toxic" contents in a way that had new meaning. An inchoate and disintegrating experience was reframed as something that could be rationally encompassed. Both the therapeutic boundaries and the patient's ego boundaries were strengthened as a result.

As I discuss in Chapter 4, projective identification reveals its dark side when it forms a major component in the progressive evolution of therapeutic boundary violations. This process starts when the therapist attempts to alleviate his or her own inner mental tensions by projecting them inappropriately onto the patient. Such a situation may be precipitated by issues that are not specifically related to the patient (e.g., a therapist who has trouble letting *any* patient leave, or a therapist who is sexually seductive with *any* physically attractive patient). Alternatively, it can occur when the therapist responds to a patient's projections with a counterprojection (*projective counteridentification* [Finell 1986]). For example, a therapist may feel impotent because he or she has internalized the patient's sense of hopelessness and worthlessness. In response, the therapist may become sexually seductive in an effort to control the patient. This involves a reversal of roles, in which the therapist attempts to have the patient become the healer.

Theories of Cognitive Development and the Development of Boundaries

It is not uncommon to observe a great deal of distorted logic employed by therapists who become involved in boundary violations. For example, Abel et al. (1992) centered their cognitive-behavioral treatment for sexually exploitive physicians around systematic efforts to correct the various patterns of faulty reasoning they observed in this population. On this basis, it might be helpful to review the phases of cognitive growth during childhood and thereby identify, in a more precise way, the developmental locus of disturbed and re-gressed thinking that occurs in the treatment situation. Although much has been added to our knowledge of cognitive development since Piaget, for purposes of clarity and simplicity, I have chosen to draw mainly upon his ideas in my discussion. Interested readers are referred to Greenspan (1992b, especially pp. 735–741) for a more comprehensive and up-to-date review of this subject.

The maturing child's ability to "know" that something is true or not true is founded on a sequential unfolding of cognitive organizers during the growth process. Piaget concluded from his experimental observations that infants in the first 6 months of life receive informa-tion as a series of sensory displays (Cobliner 1965; Piaget 1962). The discovery of "non-I," (i.e., external physical objects) proceeds grad-ually as the infant learns to visually track and reach for a toy. Piaget experimented with toys that were removed from infants' sensory fields. He discovered that they appeared to use *sensorimotor* sche-mata—such as the expectation that a rattle will make noise if it is shaken—to form the basis for their subsequent capacity to retain a permanent mental image of physical objects (Piaget 1962). A unified sense of boundary and space evolves from the coalescing of this dis-connected collection of sensorimotor schemata, and it is this process that enables a child to develop the concepts of physical substance, location, time, and causality:

> In the beginning there is not one space which contains all the objects, including the child's body itself; there is a multitude of spaces which are not coordinated: there are the buccal space, the tactilokinesthetic space, the visual and auditory spaces; each is sep-arate and each is centered essentially on the body of the subject and on actions. After a few months, however, after a kind of Copernican evolution, there is a total reversal, a decentration such that space becomes homogenous, a one-and-only space that envel-ops the others. Then space becomes a container that envelops all objects, including the body itself. (Piaget 1962, p. 123)

By experimenting with infants' ability to find hidden objects, Piaget was able to infer that by approximately 8 months of age, infants begin to retain a semipermanent mental image of a concealed toy. At this stage, infants can be seen as having acquired "permanent substance" or *object permanency* (Cobliner 1965). Piaget found that after 17 months of life, infants develop the capacity to invert the action by which a desired object has been made to disappear. In other words, infants at this age appear to possess the ability to mentally remove the screens (such as a pillow) that obscure a hidden toy. This phenomenon implies that the toy itself exists in the infant's imagination, as does the process of concealment itself.

Children ages 2–7 enter Piaget's *preoperational* stage, in which symbols such as words and pictures are differentiated from the actual objects that they represent. Children at this level of development are able to reconstruct complex behaviors. Play becomes more than an exercise—it provides a theatrical arena in which a fictional drama can be created using symbolic surrogates that represent real-life people and objects (Greenspan and Curry 1989; Piaget 1962). Children at this stage reason by configuration and by what they see. For example, if they are familiar with their neighborhood, they can retrace their steps, find a familiar place, and return back home. However, they are unable to produce a representation of this otherwise familiar path using concrete objects in a construction game (Piaget 1962). Their ability to identify the proper route to school is based on a motor memory and sensory configuration rather than on a mental representation of the whole spatial configuration. Transformations confuse children of this age. For example, if water is poured from a short, squat glass into a tall, thin glass, they are likely to think that there is more water in the taller glass. They are unable to explain where the "additional" water has come from.

From ages 7 to 11, the stage of *concrete operations* begins, during which children develop the ability to conceptualize the constancy of certain *properties* of objects such as quantity, substance, or number (Piaget 1962). The principle involved is that certain properties do not change, even if a transformation has taken place. As a result, the child begins to comprehend the generalizability and reversibility of certain operations, and to perform classification and serialized sorting based on progressively changeable properties such as size or weight. Children of this age are also able to comprehend the concept of reciprocity. For example, they now understand that the volume of liquid in a short, fat glass does not vary when it is poured into a tall, thin glass, even though it assumes a different shape. They are able to distinguish class membership from membership in a subcategory. For example, when asked to count the number of cats, dogs, and the total number of pets in a picture, they are able to correctly answer the question as to whether there or more dogs than pets, without confusing the superordinate class of "pets" with the subclassification of "cat" and "dog" (Greenspan and Curry 1989). Hartmann (1991) emphasized that this phase of development constitutes a time when latency-aged children start to "thicken" their boundaries. During latency, children begin to consolidate the ability to be industrious. This involves organizing one's time and learning to focus upon a project and to complete it.

According to Piaget (1962), the beginnings of *formal operations* do not appear until around age 12. Formal operations involve the ability to construct a hypothesis rather than relying solely on a concrete example (e.g., if A < B and B < C, then A < C) (Greenspan and Curry 1989). Adolescents are also able to entertain differing combinations of the variables that might explain a phenomenon—for example, the type of hole that a falling object will make in the ground, depending on its size, shape, weight, and speed (Greenspan and Curry 1989).

Elkind (1982) emphasized the importance of Piaget's cognitive theories in understanding the way the developing child comprehends and organizes social reality. This process may be viewed as "social cognition." He argued that Piaget's observations of the way that children develop an understanding of physical realty should also be applied to the frame of rules and expectations that constitute an important part of any social interaction, including the psychiatric treatment process. For example, Elkind emphasized that children learn best from people with whom they have formed attachments. Socialization is not merely an imitation of other people's behavior. Children also abstract from adult behavior the rules or transformations that create the behavior (e.g., prejudices). He called this process *reflective abstraction*—a form of learning that occurs by abstracting "not *from* things, but rather from a person's *action upon*

things" (Elkind 1982, p. 442); for example, a child learns about transformations by rearranging a fixed number of pennies into differing
shapes. On a social level, reflective abstraction occurs only with persons with whom there is an *emotional investment*. Internalized social
cognitions become refractory to change because they involve an underlying set of rules that follow from an emotional experience. When
formulating a therapeutic strategy for a child with behavioral difficulties, Elkind (1982) felt that it was important to investigate whether
the following problems were present:

1. Has the child been unable to learn a coherent social "frame?"
2. Is the child struggling with a social framework that he or she
   understands and rejects?
3. Is the child operating within another alternate framework that is
   sensible to him or her but is at odds with that of the child's
   environment?

The therapeutic frame provides a situation in which the patient's
emotional investment (transference) permits change through this
same process of reflective abstraction. It follows from this reasoning
that harmful distortions of the therapeutic frame can sabotage the
treatment process and foster negative social cognitions.

The therapist's ability to maintain coherent boundaries while
conducting psychotherapy is strongly related to his or her ability to
maintain mature cognitive functioning. As previously summarized in
Table 3–1, functions encompassed under the ego boundary construct
include the ability to sort, classify, and contextualize objective realities, and to differentiate them from purely mental processes. A number of factors—such as thoroughness of professional training, the
emotional stress of working with certain types of patients, and the
therapist's personal psychological problems—can have profound effects on the therapist's logical thinking. Therapists with strong narcissistic defenses against feeling unknowledgeable, helpless, or
disturbed often manifest a functional "learning disorder" that may
predispose them to commit boundary violations. For these reasons, it
is important that therapists be aware of their own tendencies to suffer
regression to less mature levels of cognitive functioning.

Greenspan and Curry (1989) emphasized that the egocentrism operating at the beginning of each Piagetian phase is correlated with an impediment toward advancing to subsequent stages of cognitive development. Their schema might be useful in pinpointing the level at which a therapist's cognitive distortions are operating. For example, these authors noted that confusion between a symbol and the thing to which it refers hampers the ability of children in the pre-operational stage (ages 2–7) from discriminating between dreams of dangerous animals and actual animals they have seen in the zoo. This concept would pertain to therapists who become confused between their fantasies about a patient and the patient himself or herself. In the stage of concrete operations (ages 7–11), Greenspan and Curry (1989) noted that the need for certainty interferes with an understanding of the concept of probability. Similarly, the fervent wish for something to be true may interfere with an acceptance of observed reality. Such problems would apply to therapists who have difficulty admitting what they do not know and who thus fail to obtain external confirmations that might dispel their cherished perceptions about a patient. Finally, Greenspan and Curry (1989) observed that an adolescent's ability to entertain and test a hypothesis is contaminated by inner perceptions and preoccupations (e.g., projecting inner concerns about intelligence or attractiveness onto other people), so that internal doubts are perceived as external criticism. Cognitive confusion stemming from this level of development might be observed in therapists who feel compelled to breach confidentiality by indiscriminately exhibiting "juicy" secrets about their patients, or who try to impress their patients with personal disclosures. "Lovesick" therapists (Twemlow and Gabbard 1989) who become romantically involved with patients probably fit into this category as well.

Boundary violations during psychotherapy are facilitated by a regression to earlier phases of cognitive development in the patient, the therapist, or both. When a patient loses his or her capacity for critical thinking and judgment, that loss is commonly a feature of the presenting disorder (e.g., psychosis, borderline personality disorder, or dissociative disorder). Even when the patient maintains superior logical and cognitive ability in daily life, he or she may regress to very archaic forms of logic within the permissive confines of the therapy.

For example, a highly functioning analytic patient may experience bizarre somatosensory phenomena, hypnoid illusions, and transient delusional phenomena in the course of free association during a session. This may be confined solely to the sessions, and evaporate as an important conscious perception as soon as the patient leaves the office. Whatever the basis of the regressive thinking, it is evident that patients are capable of using the most primitive and uncritical cognitive appraisals during psychotherapy. A patient who perceives that his or her life has meaning only insofar as the therapist defines it is in some ways like the baby who cannot maintain a permanent mental image of an object. Such patients may experience the therapist as wielding the power of life and death. Words and meaning are less important than gesture and affect. A hint of irritation or criticism in the therapist's voice can be unbearable. Such patients can be manipulated *without* words.

Patients who undergo regression as a result of either their mental disorder or the therapy process itself may function cognitively at such a level that they lack a full comprehension of class membership. These patients will accept rationalizations and explanations that would be nonsensical to most adults. They are readily placed in double binds because of their inability to understand the difference between a superordinate category and a subcategory. For example, a therapist can exploit such a patient using a method similar to that used by pedophiles to seduce children:

> It is all right for me to touch you (sexually) because I am an adult. Adults are here to protect children and tell them what to do for their own good. Therefore what I tell you is OK for you to do.

As I discuss in more detail in the next chapter, this rationalization employs a faulty syllogism. It is based on confusing the superordinate category of *all adults* with the subcategory of *beneficent adults*. The abuser deceptively (whether consciously or unconsciously) neglects to explain that there is another subcategory of adults who not only are not helpful but are in fact hurtful and exploitive to children. Such reasoning can be considered a form of bilogic. The symmetry of primary process is employed simultaneously with secondary process thinking. It is possible, in some cases, that the primary process logic is deliberately masqueraded as rational formal logic. In other situations, therapists may be caught up in the web of their own unconscious need to relieve inner tensions by projecting them onto their patients.

CHAPTER 4

Factors Common to All Boundary Violations

Let a wise man blow off the impurities of himself, as a smith blows off the impurities of silver, one by one, little by little, and from moment to moment. . . .

The fault of others is easily perceived, but that of one's self is difficult to perceive; a man winnows his neighbor's faults like chaff, but his own fault he hides, as a cheat hides an unlucky cast of the die.

If a man looks after the faults of others, and is always inclined to be offended, his passions will grow, and he is far from the destruction of passion. . . .

The Teachings of the Compassionate Buddha,
Dhammapada [The Way of Truth] XVIII[*]

A re there reliable early-warning indicators that might inform us when serious violations of the therapeutic boundaries are occurring? Most often, therapists rely on a set of formalized rules of omission and commission to identify such problems. These rules are derived from training and clinical experience. Examples include the prohibition against sexual or financial exploitation, the requirement to provide coverage in one's absence, and the principles governing maintenance of confidentiality. Rules like this are embodied both in the standards of professional behavior and in the therapist's personal ethics. They are bolstered and enforced by the therapist's conscience,

---

[*]Burtt (ed.) 1955.

by his or her desire to be professionally successful, and by his or her fear of disapproval. Sanctions might include the patient's criticism, exposure before the ethics committee of one's professional society, civil tort action, or discipline by a licensing board. In Chapters 5–13, I discuss these specific guidelines in more detail.

There are problems with presenting a list of maxims. Some are controversial because of conflicting evidence as to whether a specific behavior is beneficial or harmful, such as the appropriateness of accepting a referral from a former psychotherapy patient. Arguments over the value or harm of certain procedures can inspire fruitless contention and may even lead to the formation of new schools of psychotherapy. There are occasions when the distinction between a beneficial treatment and a boundary violation becomes quite fuzzy. An action that adversely disrupts the treatment frame in one case might conceivably be lifesaving in another. For example, it may be very appropriate to allow a suicidal patient to make special impositions on the therapist's time. Similarly, with a psychotic patient who is gripped by terrifying delusions about the therapist, it might be sensible to reassure him or her with selective disclosures about one's personal status. On the other hand, seemingly helpful and innocent deviations are often harbingers of more serious violations (R. I. Simon 1989).

Unfortunately, there is no list of procedures that would account for all permutations of the clinical decision tree. It is impossible to become engaged in meaningful psychotherapy without impinging upon the patient's psychological space in some way. Many of the more subtle types of boundary "crossings" need to be evaluated contextually before they can be deemed potentially harmful violations (Gutheil and Gabbard 1993). Therapists are faced with the conundrum of rigid codification at one extreme and relativistic looseness at the other. For this reason, examining some of the basic interactions characteristic of all boundary violations should prove helpful. The following formulation is offered as a way of organizing this problem.

The treatment boundary is a psychological containment field maintained by the therapist's mental capacity to encompass the patient's symptomatology and primary process communications. This field is essentially an extension of the therapist's own ego boundaries that have been adapted to form a professional frame of reference, or *work ego* (Rosenbloom 1992). Although the therapist's special training and society's grant of a license to practice psychotherapy support the treatment boundary, the realities of the consulting room and the temptations and stresses presented by the patient will be the ultimate test of the therapist's abilities. In the final analysis, therapists must be able to contain and modulate their own primary process thinking.

As a human being with a unique set of longings, traumatic experiences, and coping defenses, each therapist relies on his or her ego boundaries to provide an internal framework by which to organize perceptions, modulate affects, regulate impulses, and maintain a sense of meaning and involvement in relationships. Boundary violations in psychotherapy are most likely to occur when the therapist's ego boundaries have been disrupted in some way. For instance, a therapist's ego boundaries may be chronically defective because of a mental disorder such as sociopathy, psychosis, neurotic conflict, pathological narcissism, or dementia. An acute breach of ego boundaries can be triggered by general factors in the therapist's life or by the specific stress of dealing with an individual patient. General stressors might include divorce, mental illness in a relative, or financial difficulties. Stressors specific to the treatment itself might arise when the therapist attempts to treat a patient who is very attractive and seductive, who is stridently critical, or whose impulses erupt in unpredictable and alarming ways.

As I emphasized in Chapter 3, healthy ego boundaries are composed of an optimal mixture of permeability and rigidity. Permeable boundaries permit creative insight and empathy for others. A beneficial "breach" in the therapist's boundaries may occur when he or she is surprised by a discovery of something new and useful about a patient. For example, a therapist may feel wounded by a patient's sudden and unexpected criticism, yet recover by utilizing that emotional pain to empathize with the patient's internalized conflicts. On the other hand, when the breach in the therapist's ego boundaries leads to a corresponding rupture of the therapeutic frame, the therapist is at risk of becoming defensive, filled with unmodulated shame, and countercritical.

We can formulate three essential steps in the unfolding of boundary violations in psychotherapy:

1. The therapist suffers from an acute or chronic dysregulation of his or her ego boundaries. The impairment may consist of overly porous boundaries, overly "thick" boundaries, or a combination of the two.
2. The therapist employs maladaptive *intrapsychic* methods in an attempt to compensate for the impaired boundary functioning.
3. The therapist uses nontherapeutic *behavior* derived primarily from primary process reasoning in an effort to compensate for the impaired boundary functioning.

These steps are outlined in more detail in the following sections.

Dysfunction of the Therapist's Ego Boundaries

This first step in the unfolding of a boundary violation involves an impairment or weakening of the therapist's ability to maintain the caregiving role. Such a dysfunction may follow from one or more of the following factors operating singly or in concert:

Deficient knowledge.   The therapist possesses limited clinical knowledge and/or a poor understanding of the nature and function of therapeutic boundaries.

General stress or mental disorder in the therapist.   The therapist is suffering from a disruption in his or her personal life, a mental disorder that interferes with his or her ability to maintain accepted limits, or constitutionally "thin" boundaries. Examples might include therapists with acute depression, antisocial tendencies, manic excitement, schizotypal personality, or substance abuse disorder. Excessive "thinness" of boundaries may coexist with inordinate "thickness" of boundaries in therapists with narcissistic pathology or antisocial tendencies.

Treatment-induced regression.   The therapist sustains a transient impairment in his or her ability to maintain healthy ego boundaries as a result of one or more "stressors" that occur during the treatment process with a specific patient:

1. *Temptation*—The therapist perceives that the patient has entic-
   ing qualities (e.g., sexual attractiveness, social importance, valuable financial secrets, a masochistic need to be sympathetic and
   giving at any cost) that serve as a strong incentive to "bending"
   or breaking rules. These temptations serve to stir up strong feelings such as lust, envy, greed, or dependent longings. The feelings
   are intensified if the therapist notices that the patient is extremely vulnerable and defenseless—for example, a woman with
   a history of previous sexual abuse who has demonstrated her inability either to resist her attackers or to report their illegal behavior.
2. *Projective identification*—The therapist is unable to comprehend or
   contain the patient's use of projective identification. Racker
   (1957) employed the phrase "drowning in the countertransference" to describe this phenomenon. Highly suicidal or destructive patients are particularly prone to evoke such reactions in
   their therapists. In some cases, for example, fear of a patient's
   suicide becomes a chronic stressor that literally drives a therapist
   "over the edge." If the therapist cannot maintain a distinction
   between his or her own death and that of the patient, the treatment frame can be seriously endangered. With a destructive patient, the therapist might allow repeated exceptions in matters
   such as ending the session at the arranged time or timely collection of the fee because he or she is fearful of arousing the
   patient's shame or aggression. However, the therapist's fear may
   in turn reinforce the patient's sense of being a fragile and dysfunctional person who will never be capable of containing such
   negative affects. The patient's pathological frame thus winds up
   becoming the organizing principle for the treatment relationship.

The Therapist Employs Maladaptive Intrapsychic Measures to "Repair" His or Her Ego Boundaries

In this step, the loss of equilibrium precipitates a break in the
therapist's frame. In an effort to relieve the tension, discomfort, and

shame brought about by this weakening of the professional role, the therapist employs various intrapsychic mechanisms.

Deficient knowledge. The therapist uses grandiose or narcissistic defenses to deny that he or she lacks the knowledge to understand the patient's need for boundaries (see Figure 3–7). In Nathanson's (1992) terminology, this denial would constitute an "avoidance" defense against feeling shame and vulnerability. The therapist disavows reality. The same defense may be employed to deny the operation of general stress or a mental disorder. Primary process thinking (e.g., "I cannot bear to see myself as imperfect, therefore I needn't ask for help from another professional") is used as a maladaptive way of attempting to preserve a self-image of professional competence and mental stability.

General stress or mental disorder in the therapist. The   therapist who has a cognitive awareness of the boundaries begins to use bilogical thinking to reconcile the painful tension between desire and reality. For example:

> This beautiful woman (patient) isn't really that sick after all [wishful thinking]; I am a much nicer and more caring person than her abusive husband and father [possibly true but soon to become untrue]; therefore, it probably won't hurt if we become involved sexually, and will even be helpful [a faulty syllogism based on two unproven premises that are irrelevant to the conclusion].

Such thinking represents an attempt to reestablish a frame configured by the equation *I am worthwhile only when I can get desirable things for myself.*

Treatment-induced regression in the therapist. In endeavoring to be rid of the strange and discomforting tensions induced by the patient's projective identifications, the therapist regresses to primary process thinking. This regression interferes with the therapist's perception of himself or herself as a coherent person who is in control and capable of applying a professional method. A "break" has occurred in the therapist's ego boundaries that may be experienced as a profound narcissistic injury. He or she is at risk for applying bilogical thinking. For example, therapists whose ego boundaries are pathologically "thick" have an inordinate need to feel in control. As a result, they may "flood out" and be tempted to see the patient's problem—and, therefore, the patient—as an enemy that must be vanquished. Therapists with excessively "thin" boundaries may become "intoxicated" with the patient's longing for symbiotic merger.

The Therapist Employs External Methods to "Repair" His or Her Ego Boundaries

In this third and final step, the therapist attempts to regain a sense of equilibrium by using the patient to mollify his or her own discomfort.

Deficient knowledge. The therapist colludes with the patient's seductive or exploitive behavior to avoid stirring up aggression, accusations, or feelings of professional incompetence. By appeasing the patient instead of engaging with his or her distressing affects and experiences, the therapist temporarily removes the perceived disharmony.

General stress or mental disorder in the therapist. As a defense against feelings of shame, loss, abandonment, and rage, the therapist employs projective identification by externalizing these "bad" feelings of inner pain or inadequacy onto the patient. Simultaneously, the therapist may internalize the patient's desirable qualities, which the therapist perceives as missing within himself or herself. As an example of this process, Rutter (1989) outlined how a male therapist might attempt to assuage his hidden "wounds" of depression and weakness—characteristics that he perceives as unacceptably "feminine" by initiating sexual intimacy with a vulnerable female patient, who then becomes the embodiment of his own disavowed sense of injury. Such a process may also occur in nonsexual boundary violations, as illustrated by the following vignette:

Dr. Delphi was very troubled by feelings of envy and greed. She was treating Mr. Eller for depression. A wealthy, childless 84-year-old widower, he had been very dependent on his wife before she died 5 years previously. He felt that he had never contributed much to society. Over a period of several years, he had developed a strong affection for Dr. Delphi, and told her, "I don't know how I can thank you enough for the help you have given me." He suggested that one way he might be able to make an impact on the world would be to leave all of his money to her in the form of a trust fund that she could use for research and treatment of the mentally ill. Dr. Delphi readily agreed to this offer and told Mr. Eller that it would be a fitting way for him to memorialize his name after death. "It would also be a way we could maintain an enduring connection."

In this vignette, the therapist used a "bait-and-switch" tactic involving role reversal. The therapist exploited the patient's dependency, fear of death, social isolation, and loneliness by allowing him to name her as his de facto executor. In so doing, she interfered with what might have been a final opportunity to promote his autonomy. For example, she might have assisted him in dealing with the anxiety he felt about his old age and failing powers by helping him to find a way of using his wealth to make a social contribution on his own.

Treatment-induced regression in the therapist. The therapist may inadvertently act out the contents of the patient's unconscious exploitive "script" in an effort to maintain an inner sense of control. For example:

Ms. Farwah struggled with chronic self-destructive behavior that emanated from her memories of paternal incest in childhood. She projected an intense sense of helplessness and erotic arousal onto her therapist, Dr. Goode. He experienced considerable anxiety about his fantasies of sexual involvement with her. However, he was unable to acknowledge or accept how powerless he felt to relieve Ms. Farwah of her despair. He began to rationalize: "I will be saving her life by gratifying her profound sense of longing for love." He told her: "To save a life is to save the world. I can't bear for you to feel so bad; I will give you the love you never had, unlike all those bad men in your life who have hurt you and let you down. For such a desperate situation like this, the usual rules do not apply; it is all right for us to become lovers."

In this vignette, Dr. Goode unwittingly reenacted Ms. Farwah's traumatic memories. As a child, she felt that she had no choice but to submit to her father's desperate requests for sexual intercourse because he had convinced her that he needed this to stay alive.

Certain other general phenomena have been observed in the sequence of boundary violations that begins with impairment of the therapist's ego boundaries. The presence of one or more of these associated features can serve as a valuable indicator that the treatment frame is being compromised.

A Change or Slippage in the Therapist's Original Treatment Plan

Peterson (1992) viewed every boundary violation as the result of a disturbed and disconnected relationship. Such a disturbance can occur when a therapist subverts the original purpose of the treatment by turning it into something else. For example, the therapist may become intoxicated by a sense that his or her relationship with the patient is protected by a special aura or "magic bubble" (Gutheil 1989). This sense may progress to a feeling of "love" or "mystical union" similar to that experienced in a trance state. Trance logic is used to rationalize special exceptions to the therapist's accustomed way of working with his or her patients. On a primary process level, the therapist is attempting to merge with the patient. On a seemingly rational level, the changes are often justified by drawing upon the widely available eclectic smorgasbord of treatment modalities (Epstein and Janowsky 1969; Karasu 1986).

For example, a therapist who has been successfully treating a patient with psychodynamic psychotherapy begins to advise hypnosis using touch as part of the trance induction to help the patient to "relax," suggests that the sessions be conducted outside the office to increase the closeness of the relationship, or starts to accompany the patient outside the office to help with phobias or obsessions. Although the new technique might be appropriate when applied by itself as part of a coherent treatment modality, a sudden change from one type of psychotherapy to another that involves more social or physical involvement with a patient is likely to be a signal that the therapist is secretly reframing the treatment into a social relationship. Any justification that the new methods are recognized and responsible techniques may serve as a veneer of trance logic to cover forbidden wishes. For this reason, absent a clinical emergency, sudden and radical changes in treatment paradigms should be undertaken only after careful discussion with the patient, and with informed consent of the particular risk-benefit considerations involved.

Role Reversal and the Blurring of the Line Between Therapist and Patient

In his effort to become like a loving parent to his wounded patients, Ferenczi advocated the use of kisses and embraces to heal the injuries from their early trauma (Jones 1957). His "elasticity of technique" also involved allowing his patients to act as therapists for him in a form of "mutual analysis." These methods led to Freud's rebuke in 1931 (Jones 1957).

The role of therapist requires the ability to undergo, in part, a "regression in the service of the ego." In order to contain the patient's primitive conflicts, the therapist must relax his or her own ego boundaries to a certain degree. Relaxation of boundaries may progress beyond the professionally monitored treatment technique. Boundary violations begin when a blurring of the interpersonal membrane occurs that goes beyond "even-suspended attention" and empathic listening. The therapist's technique then becomes a regression in the service of the *id*. His or her observing "ego" is effectively inactivated by trance-logic tricks and self-deception. Dissolution of the capacity for self–other differentiation progresses to the point that the therapist begins to perceive the patient as a part of himself or herself (see Figure 3–7). As this experience of the patient as a "selfobject" or "mirror" becomes intensified, the ability to maintain perspective on the *transitional* quality of the treatment process is lost. The therapist temporarily or permanently loses the essence and purpose of the role of caregiver. As a result, the transitional quality of treatment as a form of "creative illusion" becomes lost. Metaphors are treated as if they are reality. This loss of perspective is a sign of a defect in the therapist's ego boundaries. It represents the beginning of a form of madness involving an increasing domination of the therapist's behavior by primary process thinking.

For many professionals who engage in boundary violations, the process often begins with a denial of the very real power differential that exists between therapists and patients (Peterson 1992). The therapist's position in relation to the patient becomes one of apparent equivalence:

> You and I are equals. I am here for you, and you are here for me.

This is a *symmetrical* statement, according to Matte-Blanco's (1988) meaning of the word, and involves the use of primary process thinking. When amalgamated with rational-sounding pronouncements, the statement becomes *bilogic:*

> Your parents didn't treat you as a full human being. Unlike them, I am here to help you learn about human respect and dignity. All people should be treated this way. I will treat you with respect. Therefore I will treat you as an equal.

This faulty reasoning involves a disavowal of the "ethos of care" and the fiduciary role so intrinsic to the act of accepting a patient for therapy. Respect is fallaciously equated with equality.

Once the boundary has been blurred to this point, the "equality" may progress to role reversal. When role reversal occurs in the treatment process, the therapist seeks a form of gratification from the patient that goes beyond the contracted fee or remunerative arrangement. Role reversal almost always involves a change from the originally stated treatment goal (Peterson 1992)—a "bait-and-switch" tactic. It is one of the key pathologic factors in the formation of a "false self" (Winnicott 1960b/1965). From the perspective of the therapist who employs projective identification to evacuate unwanted and "toxic" aspects of self, role reversal may also be conceptualized as an effort to switch from a helpless, passive position to an active one (Porder 1987). The projected affects often involve the therapist's hidden feelings of shame, envy, vulnerability, and impotence. The hidden shame is signaled by the therapist's use of "attack other" defenses such as sarcasm, teasing, ridicule, and efforts to control the patient in some way. Later on, the tragic projection comes full circle when the patient feels humiliated, exploited, betrayed, abandoned, and violated.

Ironically, when a therapist asks a patient to take care of his or her needs, things are anything but equal. In primary process thinking, however, contradictory ideas can exist side by side without conflict. The primary process thoughts might be typified by the following "symmetrical" statements in the therapist's mind:

> You and I are one . . . your needs and my needs are the same. . . . As
> I take care of you, so you should take care of me.

The irrational nature of these thoughts is more effectively concealed if the message is converted into a *bilogical* communication to the patient:

> It will be helpful for you to be considerate of others. I am another
> person; therefore, you should be considerate of me by making me
> feel good.

Double Binding

Exploitive therapists frequently use double binds to manipulate their patients. For example, a therapist might entice a patient into a sexual relationship by emphasizing how beneficial such an experience would be for the patient. At the same time, the therapist uses words or gestures to enjoin the patient from identifying the behavior as exploitive, or from revealing "their secret" to any outside party. The therapist's threats of retaliation might include rejection, abandonment, criticism, or discreditation in front of third parties (Peterson 1992). In some cases, the therapist's verbal (or nonverbal) message is imparted as follows:

> I will be psychologically destroyed by feelings of loss, abandonment, or despair if you fail to meet my expectations. You will be abandoned and it will be all your fault.

Bateson (1960) argued that double binding is cognitively toxic and psychotogenic when used as a carrier to conceal an exploitive or hostile message forced upon a vulnerable individual. The victim is usually not in a position to fight back. Double-binding messages are essentially trick communications that (on the surface at least) appear to use normal reasoning. They employ trance logic to confuse and deceive the intended victim into complying with the perpetrator's hidden intentions. Double binds work by blurring the boundaries of logical categories to create an illusion. According to Russell's theory of logical types (Bateson et al. 1956), a class is discontinuous from—and exists at a different level of logical abstraction than—its members. For example, a seductive patient might make the following statement to his or her therapist:

> I am in desperate need of a lover. Doctors are supposed to make patients feel better. Therefore you [my doctor] should relieve my need by being my lover.

This patient's logical breakdown is diagrammed in Figure 4–1. The excessive porosity of the patient's ego boundaries are reflected in his or her corresponding failure to maintain intact, logical boundaries between the two subcategories of ways that one person can help another to "feel better." Of course, the same faulty reasoning might be used by an exploitive therapist.

Double binding is regularly used by skilled attorneys in the courtroom and in the political arena to ridicule or impeach an adversary. In its most malevolent form, a double bind can be used as part of a torture designed to destroy a victim psychologically. Styron's novel

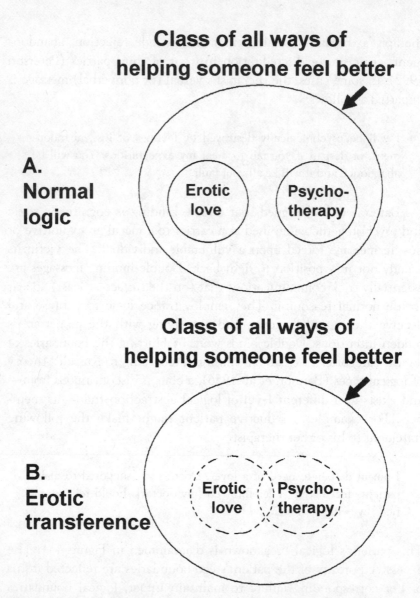

Figure 4–1. Venn diagrams comparing the faulty syllogism of a patient with an erotized transference with normal logical categorization. In rational thinking (A), "erotic love" and "psychotherapy" are logically separate sub-categories of the "class of all ways of helping someone to feel better." The erotizing patient (B) fallaciously views these subcategories of helping as being completely equivalent to one another. This situation is shown diagrammatically as a breakdown in the logical "boundaries" between "erotic love" and "psychotherapy" (*dotted portion of the circles*).

Sophie's Choice (1976) provided a fictional account of the destructive mechanism of a double bind, and the way that a perpetrator might use it to "export" his pain (via projective identification) onto a victim. In the story, Dr. Jemand von Niemand was an SS physician who was tormented because his job required that he select, among internees arriving at his concentration camp, those who were physically suitable for slave labor and those who would be immediately exterminated. His religious background was incompatible with the outrageously criminal task he was assigned. He was able, in part, to assuage this contradiction by staying continuously drunk. The beautiful heroine Sophie arrived at Auschwitz with her two children. Dr. von Niemand was attracted to her. When, in an effort to gain his sympathy, she told him that she was a Christian, Dr. von Niemand reasoned with her that, unlike the Jews who were afforded no options regarding their fate, Sophie would be granted the "privilege of a choice." He insisted that *she decide* which of her children she could keep, and which one was to be killed. With this double bind, he projected his hidden sense of shame and guilt onto Sophie. She was thereafter cursed with the irrational belief that it was she, rather than von Niemand, who was responsible for the murder of her innocent child.

Criminals frequently use a similar way of blurring logical boundaries to justify their illegal behavior. As one felon stated after being arrested:

> If the guy wouldn't have fought me when I told him to give me the money, I wouldn't have shot and killed him, and I wouldn't have been convicted of murder. Now I'm in jail because of him. He ruined my life!

In this situation, the criminal is unable to maintain the logical distinction between the hierarchy of superordinate categories and subcategories that constitute the causative factors leading to his arrest (see Figure 4–2). The victim's attempt to defend himself was a subsubcategory of those things that caused the felon's incarceration.

Some incestuous fathers also employ a blurring of logical boundaries when they attempt to ensure their children's compliance:

You are *my* daughter. You are *mine*. Therefore there is nothing wrong if I touch your genitals, since they too are *mine*.

Two very different subcategories of the concept of possession are inappropriately linked as the same (see Figure 4–3). The fiduciary possessive form "my daughter" is fallaciously equated with the exploitive possessive—"my plaything." Abel et al. (1984) reviewed seven of the most frequent cognitive distortions employed by adult offenders who seek to justify their sexual behavior with children. The pseudorational statements used by these offenders contain the formal elements of bilogical thinking, because they erroneously merge completely separate categories. For example:

Reasons why I'm in jail

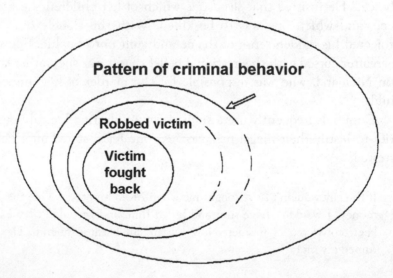

Figure 4–2. Venn diagram of a criminal's denying responsibility for his incarceration. The felon fails to acknowledge the causal hierarchy of subcategories that have resulted in his incarceration. The prime class of "reasons" is his general pattern of criminal behavior. A subset of this class is his attempt to rob this particular victim. The victim's fighting back is a sub-subset of the felon's pattern of criminal behavior. As shown by the *dotted portion of the circles*, the felon blurs the logical boundaries that would place the victim's actions in their proper position in the hierarchy.

Cognitive Distortion 7: My relationship with my daughter or son or other child is enhanced by my having sex with them. (Abel et al. 1984, 99. 100–101)

The perverted reasoning in this declaration is facilitated by the fact that the offender is able to confuse the distinction between the category of a relationship with a consenting adult and the category of a coerced relationship with a dependent child. Children who are in the preoperational phase of cognitive development (ages 2–7) are unable to muster an effective cognitive defense against an older person's faulty, bilogical reasoning.

Double binds employ the "infinitude" of primary process thinking. A part can be represented by the whole and the whole by a part. The disruption of the logical boundaries between concepts is a direct outgrowth of the perpetrator's impaired ego boundaries. Therapists

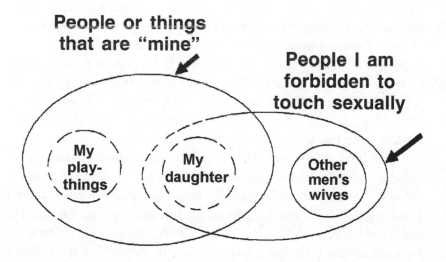

Figure 4–3. Venn diagram of an incestuous father's rationalization when sexually abusing his daughter. The incestuous father blurs the logical boundaries between "people or things" that can be considered "mine" and the class of people that are forbidden to him sexually. He tricks his daughter (and himself) by diffusing the meaning of the word "mine," and by neglecting to tell her about the existence of the other class boundaries. (The *dotted portion of the ellipse* represents the interrupted portion of the logical boundaries.)

who employ this device construct a pathological treatment frame by which they can retain a sense of meaning and involvement. For example, in the previously recounted case of Dr. Delphi, who allowed her patient Mr. Eller to name her as a beneficiary in his will, the therapist used a double bind to confuse her patient. She mixed up two different levels of meaning that were not logically comparable. Mr. Eller could easily confound his belief—"My therapist is like the whole world to me"—with his desire for a permanent tie with the therapist. He might reason, "If I want to secure my memory in the world, I must leave my money to my therapist; otherwise, I will lose this chance for an immortal (timeless) connection with her."

It is also very common for patients to employ double binds with their therapists. This behavior is derived from early experiences and is a way that they can bring their psychopathology into the treatment setting. For example, a patient who angrily criticizes the therapist for failing to offer specific advice on life decisions will later ensure that any forthcoming suggestions will be of no value, or even harmful. Such a response might result from the patient's childhood experience of being criticized as "stupid" whenever he tried to accomplish something and invariably made a trivial error. If the patient refused to try, he was called "lazy." If he tried to point out the inconsistency (i.e., to "metacommunicate"), he was called "impertinent." The therapist should try to discuss the nature and mechanism of the double bind rather than act as an enabler who becomes a victim.

Double binds are not always exploitive. When presented in an obvious and ridiculous way, they form a part of comic entertainment. Freud's (1905/1958) analysis of the way that certain jokes combine sense and nonsense can help us to understand this mechanism. He compared "joke-work" to the "dream-work" in which the requirements of civilized reasoning and the infantile impulses of the primary process are melded together for the purpose of experiencing pleasure in the face of the sometimes stuffy and onerous burdens of being civilized and responsible. In a joke, as with dreams, the most absurd concatenations of things are possible, and even desirable. The more absurd the situation, the funnier the joke is likely to be.

Many therapists recognize that double binds can be employed as part of a responsible therapeutic technique. The proper use of the mechanism involves giving a patient a logical paradox that deliberately shakes up his or her pathological frame of reference, in much the same way that Zen masters instruct their students (Bateson et al 1956; Erickson and Rossi 1979; Haley 1990). Nevertheless, therapists are cautioned that double binding can be a seductive and intoxicating way of manipulating patients with impaired ego boundaries. Systematic and continued use of therapeutic paradox runs the risk of weakening patients' ego boundaries. Double binds should be used selectively and in limited contexts, and should not be employed to feed the therapist's sense of power and control. One way of guarding against this danger is to educate the patient at some point about the mechanism and meaning of therapeutic paradoxes.

A Sense of Specialness and Entitlement

Peterson (1992) described four important themes characterizing the behavior of exploitive professionals: 1) efforts to reverse roles, 2) imposition of silence and secrecy, 3) use of double binding, and 4) indulgence of professional privilege. She emphasized that the indulgence of privilege is rationalized by a sense of entitlement and an attitude of "owning" the patient. Indulgence of privilege is one of the key features of a narcissistic, exploitive therapist who harbors a hidden agenda. Deception conceals the exploitive purpose. Exploitiveness and a sense of entitlement defend against the therapist's hidden sense of shame. By violating boundaries, the therapist is able to externalize this unbearable affect by projecting it onto the patient.

In the first phase of a serious boundary violation, such a therapist will typically idealize the patient-victim. The excitement and intensity of feeling pervading this idealization provide a strong "avoidance" defense against the therapist's hidden shame. Merger with a perfect "selfobject" offers the illusion of complete protection. During the last phase of the boundary violation, when the illusion of mystic union has become untenable, the therapist will often shift to an "attack other" defense by attempting to demean the patient as being "manipulative," "ungrateful," or "undeserving." It is at this point that the therapist discharges his or her overt feelings of shame onto the patient. The therapist may employ criticism, threats of abandonment, and warnings of retaliation to reinforce this process. In the most serious cases, therapists have been known to use threats similar to those employed by child abusers:

> No one will believe you . . . they will think you are crazy . . . I will
> have you locked up.

Exploring the sense of "projected shame" is an important task in the subsequent treatment of both violators and victims (Celenza 1991). For example, many patients who became erotically involved with a former therapist likened the experience to "sleeping with a god" (Pope and Bouhoutsos 1986, p. 92). An idealization of this intensity is not easy to argue with, often because it converges entirely with the pivotal fantasies serving to protect the patient's sense of self-worth. Sudden dismantling of their idealization may leave these patients devastated. Ulman and Brothers (1988) emphasize that the shattering of "central organizing fantasies" constitutes a key psychodynamic element in the onset of posttraumatic stress disorder. Their case of a 26-year-old incest survivor (Ulman and Brothers 1988, pp. 248–262) demonstrated that the patient's fantasy of herself as an "irresistible seductress" was a defensive effort to restore her narcissistic equilibrium. Such patients are quite vulnerable to charismatic therapists.

A therapist need not be suffering from overt narcissistic, borderline, or antisocial personality disorders to engage in serious boundary violations (see Chapter 14). Rather, the tendency may exist as a subclinical characteristic catalyzed either by the routine stress of conducting psychotherapy, or by specific qualities in a patient. Being a psychotherapist may provide a seductive gratification for an individual who has an inordinate need to feel adored and idealized. Such a therapist may resist the patient's natural progress in the treatment because that progress might lead to a replacement of idolatry with rebellion.

Therapists who as children were required to nurture an impaired caregiver are prone to be afflicted with "chronic helpfulness" (Welt and Herron 1990). This "need to be needed" is the result of narcissistic conflicts that center on having learned that one's worth and lovability depend on taking care of another person. These therapists' sense of entitlement is nurtured by their feeling that they are on a lifesaving mission of mercy. Therapists burdened with this problem are likely to have difficulty setting limits on a patient's demands, just as they were once helpless in the face of their own parents' neediness. Such therapists are prone to become enmeshed in sadomasochistic reenactments with patients who have exploitive characteristics. Out of anger that is usually based on an effort to deny a hidden sense of shame and vulnerability, a therapist may attempt to reverse roles with a patient, as if that patient were the unnurturing parent of early childhood. For example, a nurse who confessed on a popular TV talk show that she had engaged in sexual relations with one of her male patients after his discharge from the hospital explained her behavior as follows:

> I was brought up to meet other people's needs, I was trained this way since birth. I slept with a man who I took care of. . . . I would say to everyone in the helping professions, please take care of yourself! . . . I did not know who God was, I thought I could fix him, he reminded me of the man who was in my life I couldn't fix, who died because of his alcoholism. (Anonymous caller to the Phil Donahue Show, NBC TV, October 20, 1992)

Therapists who become victims often employ admixtures of "withdrawal" and "attack self" defenses against shame.

As discussed in Chapter 3, for therapists suffering from pathological narcissism, their sense of "specialness" may represent the "booby prize" that compensates for the lack of genuine acceptance experienced in early life. This "compensation"—which may take the form of money, sexual gratification, exhibitionism, or power—becomes the "everything" that fills an inner sense of "nothingness" and shame. Rebelliousness and scorn for authority are prominent characteristics seen in these individuals. They believe themselves to possess unusual gifts that entitle them to be "a law unto themselves."

Patients possessing attributes such as wealth, sexual attractiveness, fame, a need to idealize, or marked submissiveness may cause a therapist to feel "thunderstruck" by what is perceived as the precise missing counterpart that feels so necessary to fill a specific discontinuity in the therapist's own sense of self. To a person suffering from narcissistic depletion, the missing part of the self (the selfobject) *is* one's possession. That person's sense of entitlement flows from this experience of desperation. The narcissistic defense represents an effort to reconstitute a coherent inner frame of being and meaning—a way of regaining a sense of wholeness. The violated patient becomes the receptacle for the therapist's internal conflicts with shame (projective identification). When, at last, the therapist is disciplined for his or her violations, the tragic ending may also represent his or her traumatic reenactment of early feelings of mortification.

As is evident from this discussion, therapists with significant narcissistic problems are often highly refractory to education or exhortation. Narcissistic conflicts operate in this way to create a functional learning disability (see Chapters 14 and 15 for a further discussion of narcissistic pathology in therapists and educational approaches for dealing with this problem).

Specific Boundary Issues

CHAPTER 5

Introduction to Section II

It makes no difference whether it be one's roof or anything else that is dangerous and might possibly be a stumbling block to someone and cause his death—for example, if one has a well or a pit, with or without water, in his yard, the owner is obliged to build an enclosing wall ten handbreadths high, or else to put a cover over it lest someone fall into it and be killed. Similarly, regarding any obstacle which is dangerous to life, there is a positive commandment to remove it and to beware of it, and to be particularly careful in this matter . . . . If one does not remove dangerous obstacles and allows them to remain, he disregards a positive commandment and transgresses the prohibition: "Thou bring not blood." Many things are forbidden by the sages because they are dangerous to life. If one disregards any of these and says, "If I want to put myself in danger, what concern is it to others?" or "I am not particular about such things," disciplinary flogging is inflicted upon him.

Moses Maimonides (1135–1204 A.D.), *Mishneh Torah*, Hilchot Rotze'ach Ushmirat Nefesh 11[*]

The Risk-Benefit Ratio for Therapeutic Procedures

This section (Chapters 6–13) deals with specific boundary issues that serve either to protect or disrupt the treatment frame. With the exception of clearly proscribed behaviors such as violations of confidentiality, sexual involvement, or fraudulent billing, it is perilous and perhaps a bit presumptuous for me or any other author to construct a

---

[*]1944 (ann. Birnbaum); Rosner (tr.) 1986.

list of rules that would apply to the enormously complex subject of therapeutic methodology. Measures that are harmful in certain circumstances might be quite beneficial in others. Questioning specific psychotherapy techniques can also have the undesired effect of discouraging innovation. For this reason, I have endeavored to categorize an incursion across therapeutic boundaries in terms of the *relative risk* that the procedure in question will expose a patient to harm.

I do not mean to imply that we have epidemiological data available to us that could quantify this risk in terms of odds ratios and confidence levels. Nevertheless, a considerable body of clinical experience demonstrates that specific activities can lead to serious trouble. Certain behaviors, such as erotic practices with patients or deliberate financial exploitation, are damaging no matter what treatment paradigm is being employed. Adverse results can often be connected to the intrapsychic meaning that the patient ascribes to the therapist's behavior.

Because psychotherapy always involves intrusion into a patient's space, a zero-risk treatment is no more possible than a bloodless laparotomy. The concept of "boundary violation" can be compared to the "risk-adjusted" index of an investment. For any procedure, it is important to ask whether the potential gains for the patient are justified by the potential risks of injury.

What if a therapist forcibly seizes a patient who impulsively bolts out of the office screaming threats of suicide? Such an action might upset an unstable patient by stimulating fears of being controlled, assaulted, and imprisoned. If the therapist believes that the suicide threat is genuine, the danger of traumatizing the patient is counterbalanced by the necessity of saving a life. It would probably be better in this case for the therapist to act immediately and explore the patient's distressing feelings later.

In contrast, consider the case of a therapist who takes her husband's philandering cousin into psychodynamic psychotherapy after the latter has complained to her about being impotent with his most recent lover. In the absence of any emergency need for this therapist to treat a relative, the patient's interests would be better served by referring him to someone who was not a direct party to the family's problems.

In assessing risk, therapists should be aware of the potential harm both to the patient and to themselves. Careful attention to treatment boundaries offers an extra measure of protection against false accusations. As Gutheil and Gabbard (1993) have documented, cases exist in which the mere appearance of seductiveness or overfamiliarity later undermined the therapist's ability to defend against allegations of misconduct.

Aspects of Boundary Issues

In this section, five aspects of boundary issues will be considered:

Guiding principles.   Each boundary issue is organized around a set of basic verbal and behavioral statements, which are transmitted to the patient as defining messages about the therapist's trustworthiness and the nature of the treatment.

Indicated procedures.   This category refers to clinically validated forms of patient care.

Relatively risky procedures.   Behaviors fall into this category either because of clinical evidence that they are harmful in certain ways or because ongoing professional controversy exists about their usefulness or validity in the treatment setting (e.g., putting one's arm around a patient in psychodynamic psychotherapy as a way of offering comfort). For activities in this "gray area," discussion will focus on the circumstances under which such practices might become destructive to therapy, even if they are innocuous under other conditions. The fact that I have placed certain procedures into a higher-risk category does not mean that they are contraindicated or that they should be considered unethical. However, it is important that all of the risks and benefits of a procedure be weighed in any process of clinical decision making.

Contraindicated interactions.   Some activities are absolutely contraindicated because they have been shown to be almost always harmful, unethical, or illegal. An example of a contraindicated interaction is engaging in sexual activity with a current patient.

Recommended ways of dealing with specific types of boundary violations. Therapists need to recognize when they have crossed the line with a patient and take measures to repair the injury. The appropriate response will vary, depending on the type of boundary issue involved and the seriousness of the breach. Dealing with boundary violations generally involves three steps:

1. The therapist attends carefully to the patient's thoughts, feelings, dreams, fantasies, and aberrant behavior to ascertain the patient's conscious and unconscious reactions to the exploitive behavior.
2. The therapist acknowledges the way that his or her own behavior has contributed to the patient's reactions. (This should always be done in an empathic and professional way.)
3. The therapist assists the patient in dealing with the consequences of any injury that he or she has sustained. For example, the damage may involve the shattering of a fantasy, the deflation of an idealized transference, or the loss of trust in the treatment. Having faced up to the problem, the therapist is in a better position to limit the damages and to help the patient find the best solution.

If a boundary violation has caused severe harm, efforts to mend the boundaries may paradoxically increase the therapist's risk of civil or criminal exposure. For this reason, my recommendations about boundary repair *should not be used as a substitute for legal advice!* From a clinical standpoint, therapists who are able to come to their senses and recognize that they have harmed a patient are certainly in a better position to reconstitute the therapeutic relationship than would be the case if they continued to deny that any problem existed. Save perhaps for the most serious types of exploitation, it is rarely too late to try to assist one's patient by acknowledging the violation and helping him or her to understand its psychological consequences. Although the patient is likely to experience feelings of having lost an idealized caregiver and of being betrayed, it may nevertheless be the first time that anyone in the patient's life has had enough insight or personal coherence to own up to such an error, and to offer help in repairing the damage.

From a legal aspect, however, "confessions" are like rolling dice. Often, patients who have been abused are already quite familiar with the tears and pleas for forgiveness that follow exploitive behavior. They may look upon any confession with cynicism and mistrust. Some may view a therapist's admission as an opportunity to counterexploit. For these reasons, therapists who think they have committed a *serious* boundary violation are advised to seek legal counsel, personal psychotherapy, and supervision with a senior colleague before blindly following any of the advice in this book. Personal psychotherapy is particularly important, because therapists who have committed serious violations may be suffering from treatable psychopathology (see Chapter 14). Their problems may involve denial and repetitive, self-defeating behavior. Therapists need to reconstitute their personal ego boundaries before they can attempt to fix a damaged treatment. An emotional outburst of "true confession" with a confused and angry patient is likely to compound the latter's problems and to increase the therapist's legal exposure.

Defining boundaries can be experienced as befuddling, frustrating, and even demeaning by many patients. To foster trust, the therapist must proceed in a sensitive and respectful way. For this reason, in this section I employ clinical vignettes to illustrate various ways of helping patients to understand the purpose for the limits we as therapists must sometimes enforce.

CHAPTER 6

Stability: Creating an Atmosphere of Trust and Reliability

The shifts of Fortune test the reliability of friends.

Cicero, *De Amicitia*, XVII

Guiding Principles for Establishing a Stable Therapeutic Setting

Trusting relationships are built on predictability and reliability. It is hard to put one's faith in a person or situation that is erratic, unpredictable, or filled with unpleasant surprises. As mentioned in Chapter 2, a patient's willingness to open up will depend on the therapist's ability to maintain a grip on his or her own madness (Langs 1984–1985b).

The principle of stability is an ideal. No therapist can be totally consistent. He or she might miss a session because of illness in the family without having an opportunity to notify the patient beforehand. Mechanical problems with an automobile could prevent the therapist from coming to a session on time. An emergency call from another patient might necessitate interrupting a session in progress. Life is filled with the unpredictable. Although it is not possible for the therapist to be perfect, he or she must understand how intensely

119

dislocating this kind of experience can be for patients. It is also valuable for a patient to learn that the therapist is concerned about his or her reaction to unexpected changes in the treatment setting. If the therapist can handle these situations in an empathic way, the patient receives an important defining message:

> My therapist is going to a lot of trouble to provide a safe and consistent place for me to talk with him or her. Even when things change, my therapist wants to know how these changes have affected me. He or she is a committed, reliable, and steady person who is interested in how different things might upset me. This is a place where I might be able to expose and explore the irrational stuff inside me.

Indicated Ways of Maintaining Consistency and Stability

Establishing a treatment contract.   Any collaborative endeavor must begin with certain defining agreements between the participants. In psychotherapy, the contractual arrangement forms the basis for the working alliance between patient and therapist. The treatment contract is initiated when the patient is able to accept the therapist's diagnoses and treatment recommendations. The therapist should reframe the patient's problem in a way that is both cognitively and emotionally meaningful. He or she should also present the risks and alternatives to the proposed treatment plan, and should advise the patient how to get the most out of it (see the discussion of informed consent in Chapter 8). Other important components of the working agreement include the schedule for time and location of appointments, provisions for emergencies, and arrangements for the payment of fees. When coherently defined, these administrative arrangements become an integral part of the stable therapeutic frame. Discussion of these issues empowers the patient to participate as an active collaborator in the therapeutic process.

Most therapists establish contractual arrangements in an informal way during the first few visits with a patient. Others employ formal written agreements. Some patients find a highly structured contract reassuring, particularly those who were raised in very chaotic families. Whatever method is used, it is essential to take these agreements very seriously. For a stable and effective treatment to proceed, a breach by either party should be addressed immediately.

Herman (1992b) advised that therapists specifically encourage the principles of truthfulness, full disclosure, and collaboration when establishing a treatment contract with chronically traumatized patients. Abused individuals burdened by prolonged exposure to an atmosphere of deception and secrecy need to be informed that treatment cannot be effective without a commitment to honesty. I believe Herman's advice to be valid for *all* psychotherapy patients, because it is not always obvious at the outset if a patient has been nurtured in an environment framed by distortions and lies. Treatment is easily destroyed if the patient consciously deceives the therapist. Depriving the therapist of vital clinical information can even result in the patient's death.

Demonstrating one's commitment to regularity, consistency, and punctuality. At the risk of sounding simplistic—somewhat like telling airline pilots not to crash planes into mountainsides—I want to emphasize how important it is just for the therapist to show up. It is easy to become so caught up in the complexity of our work that we forget how sensitive some patients can be to even the most trivial lapses with regard to lateness, absences, and erratic scheduling. Many patients have endured a childhood that was seriously marred by capricious and unpredictable behavior on the part of their caregivers. For this reason, therapists should attempt to provide as much regularity, punctuality, and consistency of location as possible. Such efforts lay the foundation for a stable treatment frame—one that promotes the patient's sense of security, trust, and reliant expectancy. Even when departures from this ideal are necessary from a practical standpoint, most patients seem to sense and appreciate the therapist's level of commitment to this goal.

Similarly, finishing sessions at the appointed time helps to establish an atmosphere of appropriate limits and seriousness of purpose. In certain situations, such as often occur with patients who are self-destructive or who have multiple personality disorder, the therapist can find it very difficult to end sessions as scheduled. Obviously, clinical flexibility is required in this regard. Discussing the issue with the patient can assist in structuring a coherent arrangement that has a "predictable" variability. For example, the patient can be asked to share in the responsibility by scheduling in advance for extra sessions (or longer sessions) at times when he or she perceives that clinical exigencies require this.

Discouraging interruptions. It is important to maintain the "sanctity" of the patient's time by configuring an office arrangement that discourages intrusions and precludes the need to answer phone calls during sessions. Provisions should be made for distinguishing between emergency and routine calls, either by using a pager or an emergency phone line or by having secretarial staff screen calls. Colleagues and staff should not be allowed to interrupt sessions unless the matter is truly urgent.

Providing advance notice of absences. Patients should be given as much advance notice as possible when the therapist expects to miss a session.

Ensuring coverage for patient emergencies during one's absence. Therapists need to instruct patients about how to reach them in an emergency. Determining the existence of an emergency should be the *patient's* responsibility; it should not be decided by the answering service or the therapist. If the therapist believes that a patient is starting to abuse this prerogative, it is probably best to handle the situation as an urgent matter in the acute phase, and wait for a more propitious time to discuss self-defeating or manipulative aspects of the patient's behavior (see Chapter 13). Therapists should ensure that their practice is covered by a competent colleague when they are unavailable for emergencies during evenings, weekends, or vacations. Care for a patient enrolled in psychotherapy is not limited to the time during sessions: rather, it should be viewed as taking place 24 hours per day and 365 days per year.

Maintaining a consistent therapeutic demeanor.   The therapist's behavior and therapeutic method should be as consistent as possible to reduce the elements of surprise and uncertainty.

Maintaining consistency as to who participates in the treatment. Some consistency should be maintained as to who the actual participants of the therapy will be. Aside from collateral interviews with family members at the beginning of treatment or special indications such as crisis intervention, it is generally best not to allow shifting participation from a family therapy paradigm to individual therapy or vice versa. I have observed many patients (who have been referred for subsequent psychotherapy) whose previous treatment was derailed by a mixed or erratic treatment paradigm. The most common pattern usually involves a therapist who started individual psychodynamic therapy with a patient but, after seeing the patient's spouse for several collateral or couples psychotherapy visits, proceeded to take the spouse into parallel individual treatment. A shift of this kind tends to interfere with maintaining a stable treatment paradigm and may place the therapist in a role conflict between the two spouses (see Chapter 7).

Many therapists successfully employ a family systems approach in conjoint family therapy conducted with two or more related individuals. In these situations, allowing one family member to be absent from any of the sessions is quite risky in that such a practice violates the original agreement that problems will be addressed in a conjoint setting. Attempting to temporarily shift from a conjoint paradigm to individual treatment is dangerous because one or more of the family members who have been "left out" may perceive discussions during their absence as a misappropriation of their communications. This is particularly true in couples therapy when the missing spouse has deliberately absented himself or herself from a session. Behavior of this kind may be a way of "testing" the therapist's resolve. For example, a man who is suspicious of his wife might "miss" one of his couple psychotherapy sessions to see if the therapist can be trusted not to "steal" his wife. For this reason, when using a family paradigm with two conjugal partners, it is inadvisable to allow one spouse to come alone. In my own practice of couples psychotherapy, I carefully explain this policy in advance, including the fact that the couple will be billed for a missed session should one of the partners be unavailable. In addition, should one partner be late, I do not let the other start the session alone. When treating a multigenerational family group, it may be reasonable to take a more flexible stance if children of the conjugal pair are late or absent.

Some psychotherapeutic methods successfully employ a mixed paradigm of individual and collateral family involvement. This is best done in a structured way that is designed from the outset as a part of the treatment plan. For example, Network Therapy for patients who abuse alcohol (Galanter 1993) might employ individual sessions augmented by communications with a spouse. The spouse is not considered the index patient but might be expected to inform the therapist if the patient neglects to take his or her disulfiram.

Relatively Risky Procedures Regarding the Maintenance of Consistency

When significant breaches of treatment stability occur, patients often interpret them as a sign that the therapist is a disorganized or incoherent person who has difficulty dealing with chaotic phenomena. Such breaches constitute hazard signals to patients who are struggling with the confusing and frightening internal stimuli of mental disorders or with stressful life situations. Patients who are upset by a therapist's inconsistencies will sometimes complain overtly about the therapist's lack of consideration. More often, however, their reaction is an unconscious one and is revealed in the form of free associations, dreams, or acting-out behavior.

For example, a patient might start to miss sessions or come late in response to similar behavior on the part of the therapist. Such behavior may be an unconscious form of retaliation. It is important for the therapist to be alert to these issues in order to account for unexpected therapeutic impasses (Kluft 1992). Without an awareness of such phenomena, the therapist will find it difficult to take appropriate corrective action.

Contraindicated Reactions to Issues Concerning Stability

Failing to attend to a patient's signals. Therapists must attend to their patients' overt and covert efforts to deal with instability in the treatment setting.

Reacting defensively to a patient's complaints. A therapist should avoid justifying his or her behavior or criticizing the patient in response to the latter's complaint about the therapist's unreliability. Many therapists have a hard time with stability/consistency issues because they experience a focus on such details as a form of "obsessive rigidity" or "imprisonment." These therapists prefer a looser style and tend to disparage patients who complain about their erratic behavior:

> Mr. Adams complained to his therapist Dr. Brown because she was frequently 5–10 minutes late in starting the sessions.
>
> Mr. Adams told his therapist: "It makes me furious that you are always coming late. You charge me for the time if I am late, but I am not allowed to dock you when you waste my time!"
>
> Dr. Brown responded: "Look here, I have a very busy schedule and many matters to attend to. You should be realistic about things like this and realize that it just isn't possible to always start on time. Besides, why should you worry about when we start? You are out of work and don't have anything else to do anyway."
>
> Mr. Adams felt hurt and demeaned by this response. He believed that Dr. Brown was telling him that she was more important and worthwhile a person than he. He felt ashamed that he had not been able to get a job.

Stability does not mean setting one's watch by the Naval Observatory or fanatically insisting on perfection; rather, it refers to being aware of one's own rhythms and those of the patient. As with the "good enough" caregiver of early childhood, maintaining homeostasis requires careful attention to the way disruptions can upset one's patients and interfere with their ability to cooperate with and benefit from the treatment process.

Recommended Ways of Dealing With Boundary Violations Pertaining to Stability

Covert signs of stability violations. The patient becomes preoccupied with dreams of abandonment and rejection; these may include being thrown out of windows, kicked off a bus, or denied entrance to a theater. The patient has fantasies of wanting to reject or abandon others. The patient blames himself or herself for letting others down, but this self-reproach is not commensurate with the patient's actual behavior. The patient talks about people in his or her life who don't care, or who "let him [or her] down." The patient starts missing sessions or coming late after a pattern of regular attendance. The patient abruptly announces a desire to drop out of treatment.

Reparative responses. If a therapist suspects a problem with stability in the treatment setting, he or she should try to identify the specific issue and explore it with the patient. With some patients, it may be a question of them needing a regular appointment at the same day and time instead of one that varies from week to week. He or she may also need more frequent visits. Other patients may be unable to deal with the therapist's chronic lateness or tendency to take phone calls during sessions. If the therapist cannot correct such problems, it may be best to refer the patient to another therapist with whom there will be a better "match" rather than burden the patient with the shame of thinking that he or she "should learn to be more flexible." Some patients cannot trust a therapy that lacks a certain level of predictability. If they didn't have this problem, they might not have needed to come for treatment in the first place.

C H A P T E R   7

Whom Should a Psychotherapist Treat? Problems of Patient Selection When a Dual Relationship Exists

To do two things at once is to do neither.

Publilius Syrus, *Sententiae*, 7

Guiding Principles for Patient Selection and Referrals

In any relationship between two people, a potential conflict may arise between mutuality and self-interest. A patient is best served by a therapist who offers help that has an acceptably low risk of causing harm. Although a psychotherapist needs patients in order to pursue a professional practice and earn a living, he or she also has a fiduciary responsibility to guard against any conflict of interest that might sabotage treatment. Because a second agenda is likely to interfere with treatment efficacy and thereby harm the patient, therapists

127

should avoid entering into dual relationships with patients. In so doing, the therapist communicates the following behavioral message:

> I am going to avoid any competing interests that might interfere with the commitment I have made to try to help you. I will be here for *you*.

In a national survey of American psychologists, Pope and Vetter (1992) found that 17% of their respondents reported ethically troubling incidents that fit within the category of "blurred, dual, or conflictual relationships." One type of dual relationship arises when the therapist has a prior nontherapeutic connection with the patient, such as consanguinity, social involvement, or business dealings. Dual relationships may be unavoidable in certain social and community contexts, and a clinical risk-benefit appraisal must be adjusted accordingly. For example, suppose that a therapist who lives in a remote rural area offers psychotherapeutic crisis intervention to a neighbor. The fact that this decision takes place in a rural setting does not make it less risky for the patient, but the risk-benefit ratio might be more acceptable because a greater chance exists that no alternate therapist is available. A similar situation would hold for a psychotherapist who serves a small ethnic or religious community of which he or she is also a member. Opportunities to make viable referrals to another therapist might be quite constrained in such a situation. The fact that the risk-benefit appraisal might weigh in the favor of starting treatment despite the presence of a dual relationship in these limited circumstances should not be used to rationalize that such relationships are acceptable in *all* situations, just as the more lax standards of emergency first aid in the field do not change the requirements for aseptic procedures in the operating room.

It is worth remembering that there are many patients whose capacity to make gains in therapy is quite tenuous, often as a result of having suffered incoherent and disruptive relationships in childhood. Helping such patients is difficult even under the best of circumstances. By attempting to treat them in a dual-relationship situation, the therapist might sabotage their already limited opportunities for improvement.

A restriction on accepting patients is not easy for most therapists to accept. Of the 532 psychiatrists who responded to our survey, 84% indicated that they had accepted individuals for psychotherapy who were known to be referred by current or former patients (Epstein et al. 1992). In a highly competitive field in which treatment referrals are equated with economic survival, there is a strong incentive to minimize the concern that harm will befall patients, especially when the dual relationship appears to be a trivial one. Nevertheless, therapists increase the risk of adverse treatment response when they attempt to treat patients with whom they have had prior nontherapeutic contact. Included in this category are acquaintances, friends, family members, and referrals from other patients. The motivating factor in the referral process should be the patient's need for the most suitable therapist. The referral source should not subject the patient to unnecessary risk or to preventable conflict of interest that might sabotage the treatment. Economic factors should not really have to play so important a role in refusing patients because of dual relationships. A respected colleague with whom the therapist has a cross-referring relationship is likely to have just as many conflicts with his or her own referrals. If clinicians handle the problem by sending high-risk referrals to such colleagues, the net "referral loss," averaged over time, will approach zero.

Indicated Ways of Accepting Patients

Referrals from sources with low risk for causing dual-agency conflicts. There are many referral sources that have very low potential for producing a dual-agency conflict between therapist and patient. Although it is impossible for me to provide a complete list, such sources generally consist of recommendations from other professionals and institutions or of patients' own efforts in finding the therapist's name from directories, publications, public lectures, or advertisements. In my view, the determining factor in this regard is that the referring source should not have a preemptive or special fiduciary connection *with both the therapist and the patient* that has a reasonable possibility of placing the therapist in an unresolvable conflict of loyalties. For example, a therapist should not agree to treat his or her own brother's boss. There is simply too much potential for such an arrangement to lead to serious problems between the therapist and the boss, between the boss and the therapist's brother, and between the therapist and his or her brother.

Relatively Risky Referral Sources

Current or former patients.   The topic of patient referrals is like a minefield because it is so controversial. Evidence that accepting referrals from current or former patients is a risky procedure is far from established and is based largely on clinical observations. I have decided not to avoid discussing this issue because I believe that whatever a clinician's point of view in this regard, he or she should certainly be aware of the potential hazards involved.

Many responsible and highly competent therapists accept referrals from patients. These therapists reason that as a satisfied customer, their patient is in the *best position* to make a referral to a friend or relative. In providing such a recommendation, the patient can help another person obtain a good therapist while also expressing gratitude for his or her own improvement. Although this reasoning sounds intuitively correct and is certainly in keeping with the way every other clinical and nonclinical profession seems to operate, I have problems with these arguments because I have seen too many cases in which such reasoning led to serious problems for one or both patients involved.

Accepting referrals from current and former patients can lead to unresolved therapeutic issues for both patients. This practice probably has more risk of creating difficulties for the patient who gives the therapist's name to a friend or acquaintance than for the new patient who receives it. Accepting such referrals is also more likely to lead to serious deviations in the treatment frame for *current* patients who give out the therapist's name than for *former* patients who have long since terminated treatment.

It is certainly possible that no harm whatever will result for either patient, but this does not relieve the therapist of the responsibility of making a clinical judgment in this regard. Because investigating the underlying issues can be quite difficult, my own practice when patients are referred to me in this manner is to recommend another therapist. Depending on the nature of the circumstances, I either handle this over the telephone or see the new patient for a single consultation in order to assist me in making the best recommendation.

Langs (1973) advised that any reservations in a clinician's mind regarding the appropriateness of a referral should be resolved in favor of referral to a colleague. He argued that patient referrals often represent an effort on the part of the original patient to seduce, demean, or act out with the therapist. Langs (1973) cited a number of underlying factors that might motivate a referring patient to present the "gift" of a referral to his or her therapist (see Table 7–1).

Patients who refer friends or relatives to their former therapist may be trying to reestablish contact through a surrogate. Although such patients may consciously believe they are being altruistic, often an unconscious purpose is at work that needs to be identified and

Table 7–1.   Possible unconscious factors motivating a patient to refer a new patient to his or her therapist

- An effort to assuage guilt over aggressive fantasies or behavior aimed at the therapist.

- An attempt to offer a surrogate as a way of allaying conflicts over the wish to escape from therapy.

- A wish to seduce the therapist into a closer involvement, either in a sexualized or a dependent manner.

- A need to repeat and act out sibling rivalry conflicts.

- A need to repeat and act out incestuous oedipal fantasies.

- A need to disavow an impending separation from the therapist, whether it be a vacation or an anticipated termination of the treatment.

- For former patients, an effort to test the integrity of the therapist by promoting his or her betrayal, a mutual acting-out, or the sabotage of a previously successful treatment.

Source. Adapted from Langs 1973, pp. 60–62.

discussed rather than enacted in reality. The therapist may inadvertently foster problems for both patients if he or she accepts this "proposal" without further investigation.

The former patient's inappropriate way of "holding on" to the therapist may also involve voyeuristic fantasies. He or she will often question the new patient about what the therapist did or said:

Mrs. Cabot terminated therapy with her therapist Dr. Dunn after having experienced significant improvement in her depressive symptomatology. Dr. Dunn had been treating her with imipramine and supportive psychotherapy. She disagreed with Dr. Dunn's suggestion that it might be worth staying in therapy a while longer to explore her sensitivity to rejection and her fears of being perceived as unattractive. Eight months later, Mrs. Cabot told her friend, Ms. Earl, that Dr. Dunn was a "miracle worker" who would surely help her with her substance abuse, impulsiveness, and promiscuity.

Ms. Earl was an extremely attractive young woman and intellectually gifted. Dr. Dunn readily accepted Ms. Earl into psychotherapy. After her first visit, she went back to her friend Mrs. Cabot and thanked her for the referral, informing her: "You were right about Dr. Dunn, he is very warm, friendly, and understanding, I think we are going to get along very well!"

Several weeks later, Mrs. Cabot developed the sudden onset of severe aphthous stomatitis for the first time, and suffered a relapse of her depression. She became suicidal and cut her wrists. She was hospitalized as a result, and told the admitting psychiatrist, Dr. Faust, that she had felt a deep sense of shame and inadequacy about herself since childhood, and a sense of betrayal by her parents, who favored her younger sister who was so good-looking and talented. She also told Dr. Faust that she was preoccupied with her friend Ms. Earl, whom she felt possessed all of the attributes of beauty and intelligence that she herself lacked. Mrs. Cabot did not want Dr. Dunn to be called into her case—she felt that he would be disappointed in her because she had gotten worse.

In this vignette, there was a strong indication that the original patient felt betrayed when Dr. Dunn took her attractive friend into therapy. She reenacted the trauma of her childhood with Dr. Dunn and her friend in a manner that mirrored the way her parents had favored her younger and seemingly more appealing sister. It should be remembered that in the unconscious mind, time has no relevance. Transference towards a "former" therapist may be invested with the full force of emotion, even many years after the last visit. As Hall[*] (cited in Gonsiorek and Brown 1990, p. 291) has stated, "The half-life of transference exceeds that of plutonium." Adherence to the principle of avoiding dual agency would have prevented this type of problem. When a therapist agrees to treat a patient, he or she assumes a serious responsibility. Competent therapy requires an enduring commitment to the patient's well-being. For this reason, therapists should assiduously avoid putting themselves in situations that have high potential for conflicting interests.

An even more complicated scenario might have evolved if Mrs. Cabot had decided to return to Dr. Dunn, thereby exposing both patients to the risk of acting out sibling rivalry issues in their therapy. Although such events are often considered "grist for the mill" in treatment, it becomes harder for the therapist who has actively participated in constructing such a situation to credibly work with the patient on the problem. Attempts to treat the spouse of a patient in current individual therapy, or scheduling individual sessions with one spouse of a pair in couples psychotherapy with the same therapist, will often result in similar problems of jealousy, mistrust, and destructive behavior. The treatment will often be disrupted, sexual acting-out may occur, and marriages may break up before the therapist has any real opportunity to clarify the feelings involved or to help the situation.

The next vignette illustrates the potential problem for the patient who is being referred, and how the therapist can handle this type of situation in a way that protects both patients from unnecessary risk:

> Mr. Gordon was a 40-year-old married man who sought treatment because of agoraphobia and panic attacks. As a child, he was overstimulated by an aggressive, domineering, and seductive mother.

---

[*] Original reference not available.

His father was passive and distant. After approximately 2 years of psychotherapy combined with medication, his anxiety symptoms had markedly improved. He began to develop intense erotic fantasies about women other than his wife and impulsively initiated an extramarital affair. His therapist, Dr. Helms, questioned whether he might be acting out unconscious sexual feelings toward her (the therapist), feelings that might be linked to forbidden wishes to possess and dominate his mother, wishes that might also serve as a way of switching from the passive to the active position. Mr. Gordon agreed that he sometimes had passing sexual thoughts about the therapist, and conceded that he often wished he could turn the tables on his mother.

However, he argued that his new girlfriend made him feel alive in a way that he had never experienced before, and that he wasn't going to give her up. Furthermore, he resented what he perceived as the therapist's effort to interfere with his newfound sexual freedom. Despite Dr. Helms' efforts to maintain a neutral and exploratory position, the patient dropped out of treatment.

Approximately 1 year later, Dr. Helms received a call from a Mr. Irving, who asked for an appointment. He told her that he had been in treatment with Dr. James, who was retiring from practice, and that he was looking for a new therapist. Since Dr. James had occasionally referred to Dr. Helms in the past, she mistakenly assumed that he was the referral source. Mr. Irving—a handsome, well-groomed, and very charming man in his early 40s—arrived promptly for his appointment. He stated that he was a successful businessman. Dr. Helms noticed that she felt an immediate attraction to him.

On questioning Mr. Irving about his prior therapy, it became clear that he had in fact been referred by the former patient Mr. Gordon, who had given a glowing recommendation of Dr. Helms. Mr. Gordon had been his college roommate and they used to drink and go on double dates together. Mr. Irving complained of problems with self-esteem and a sense of emptiness. Despite his many relationships with women, he was always disappointed and was unable to achieve a sense of closeness with any of them. His parents had separated when he was 14. An only child, his mother treated him as special, and would often have him act as a "go-between" and confidante for her numerous extramarital affairs. This occurred while she and his father were still together. After his parents' divorce, his mother took up with a series of men and seemed to lose interest in him. His sense of emptiness appeared to commence during that period in his life. He told Dr. Helms that he would like her to take his case for psychotherapy.

Although Dr. Helms was interested in working with this articulate and appealing patient, and had plenty of open time available to see him, she felt a sense of uneasiness about his prior connection with Mr. Gordon. She was particularly disturbed by his history of having been used as a surrogate by his mother to take messages to her boyfriends, and by the possibility that he was being used by Mr. Gordon in the same way. She did not immediately rule out taking his case, but decided to explore the psychodynamic issues with him and to outline the risks that entering treatment with her might entail.

She told Mr. Irving: "You tell me that another patient who has been to see me has given you my name. This presents some potential problems that I would like to discuss with you before either of us makes a decision about whether I would be the best person to be your psychotherapist or whether it might be better for me to refer you to someone else. First of all, I can't confirm or deny that I know this other person you are talking about, because confidentiality dictates that I keep my mouth shut when it comes to somebody that walks in here to consult with me. However, without getting into the issue of what I know or don't know about any other person, we can limit our conversation to the information that is already available to you. Although it is not necessarily a contraindication, a psychotherapy referral from a friend to his or her own therapist, past or present, can in some circumstances pose a problem for treatment. To take a hypothetical example, one patient might refer a friend and then there could be complications because of fear that the therapist is discussing the other's case. In other situations, there might be feelings of jealousy and rivalry because the two patients start comparing their sessions."

"Oh don't worry about that, Doctor Helms," Mr. Irving assured her, "Mr. Gordon told me he now goes to someone else, and has no plans to return to you, besides which, I would never tell him what we talk about."

Dr. Helms replied: "People have been known to change their

minds about whom they see for therapy, so it's important to think about whether you want to take a chance about that. There are other therapists, who are just as competent as I, with whom this whole thing would not be an issue. But even if rivalry or comparing notes never became a factor, there's something else I wanted to ask you about. You told me that as a child your mother employed you as a messenger for her own purposes. Being her confidante was a way you could hold on to her and get her attention and approval, even though it was upsetting for you to have to keep secrets from your father. Do you think this might be similar to what you have been telling me about your relationship with your friend?"

At this point Mr. Irving said: "What you were just talking about reminded me of the fact that Mr. Gordon always used to get me to scout things out for him with the girls he was interested in. I would always do it, even though I didn't like it, because I wanted him to like me. In fact, in one situation in college I went out with one of his former girlfriends because he suggested it, and he wanted me to tell him all about our sexual relationship. I wish you could be my doctor, but maybe you are right about my thinking twice about it. I think maybe you should give me the name of another therapist, as you mentioned; that way I'll have someone who's just there for me."

Five years later, Mr. Gordon called Dr. Helms for consultation. He had obtained a divorce from his first wife and had entered into a stormy relationship with his girlfriend. She had become insanely jealous and possessive of him and would become physically and verbally abusive when she thought he was looking at other women. Couples therapy with her was ineffective. He had recently broken up with her because her behavior had become intolerable.

Afterwards, he began to experience a recurrence of his anxiety symptoms. He remembered that Dr. Helms had previously been a solid and reliable presence in his life and he wanted to come back so that he could work on his problems. He remembered her way of handling the referral with Mr. Irving. He was a little puzzled about it at the time, but he now looked at it as a sign of her being a very careful person. It made him admire and respect her all the more.

In this vignette, the therapist was able to avoid inadvertently facilitating the exploitive acting-out of the first patient and the masochistic tendencies of the second. She successfully protected the first patient's confidentiality and was able to provide a useful evaluation and referral for the second.

Relatives of a patient in individual therapy.   Treating the spouse of a present or former patient is a variant of other types of patient referrals because it involves two preemptive relationships—that between the referring patient and the therapist, and that between the referring patient and his or her spouse. Dahlberg (1970) presented nine case histories involving therapist-patient sex. In two of the cases, the offending therapist had also independently treated the patients' husbands. In a third case, the therapist married his female patient after initiating intercourse during treatment. When she required additional therapy, he referred her to his former training analyst but insisted that she not tell the analyst that they had met while she was his patient. The therapist made the decision to send his wife-patient to his former analyst because he knew that she (the wife) would be afraid to injure his reputation with an important colleague. He also figured that even if his wife did "spill the beans," his former analyst would be loath to expose him. The analyst agreed to accept her for treatment and did not learn the truth until several years later, when the couple divorced.

Whenever a therapist attempts to treat the spouse of a patient who has been in ongoing individual psychotherapy, all parties become burdened by an unnecessary conflict of interest. Such an arrangement also increases the risk of an adverse outcome. Without the possibility of full disclosure and the trust of confidentiality, the therapeutic frame cannot be configured as an effective "holding" environment.

The therapist's own friends or relatives. A serious problem arises when therapists attempt to treat individuals with whom they currently have—or formerly had—a personal relationship. The most glaring example of this situation is seen when a therapist employs psychotropic medication, hypnosis, or psychodynamic interpretations with members of his or her own family. Although treatment of family members is a very common phenomenon, it is a risky practice that impedes objective therapy and can lead to iatrogenic disorders. La Puma and Priest (1992) reviewed some of the issues arising when physicians attempt to treat members of their own families. Problems include incomplete examination, the difficulty of maintaining objectivity, and an impairment in the usual doctor-patient relationship (i.e., "familiarity breeds noncompliance") (La Puma and Priest 1992).

Winchell (1992) emphasized that physicians who prescribe for family members should not mislead themselves into thinking that they are relieved of the responsibility of maintaining the usual standards of care, such as keeping medical records, performing physical examinations, and obtaining laboratory tests. In one case that Winchell reviewed, a physician was reprimanded by the Maryland state licensing board because he continued to prescribe narcotics for his wife. Despite his contention that he was trying to rescue his wife when no one else seemed to be helping her, the licensing board found that this physician had lost his medical objectivity and was being manipulated into enabling his wife's substance abuse.

Spouses and children who have been "treated" by a therapist-relative frequently complain of feeling confused and violated. When seen in subsequent psychotherapy with a nonrelative, they are often very mistrustful of the treatment process because they have experienced it as a form of manipulation and control. It is not uncommon for these patients to employ terms like "mind control" or "being brain-fucked" to describe the intrusive, but ostensibly well-meaning efforts of their clinician relatives. In our study (Epstein et al. 1992), 79% of the respondents acknowledged making diagnoses or psychodynamic formulations with their own family members or social acquaintances. Using factor analysis, we discovered that this behavior correlated with feeling gratified by a sense of power when controlling patients' behavior through advice, medication, or behavioral restraints.

Other persons having a prior nontherapeutic relationship with the therapist.   For the same reasons mentioned above, therapists should avoid treating employees, acquaintances, or other persons with whom they are likely to have regular dealings.

Forensic patients. A potentially serious conflict of interest is created when a therapist attempts to treat a patient who has been referred for forensic purposes in cases where the professional has already
testified, or plans to testify, in a legal proceeding on the patient's
behalf. Forensic testimony requires extensive collateral investigation
that can be intrusive and antitherapeutic. The jarring shift of roles
from therapist to forensic expert, or vice versa, can be humiliating
and highly traumatic for the patient. Testifying about a patient in
current treatment tends to stir up reality-based fantasies about the
therapist's role as a savior. If the patient wins the legal case, expectations are raised about the therapist's magical powers. The therapist's
real (psychotherapeutic) powers are likely to be devalued forever-
more. On the other hand, if the patient loses the legal case, there is a
good chance he or she will blame the therapist, no matter how irrelevant the therapist's testimony might have been to the outcome.

This caveat does not apply to those rare situations when the
therapist is called as a "fact" witness about some specific event rather
than as an expert who renders opinions about findings. Being called
to testify as to facts might occur when it is necessary for the therapist
to certify that a patient has attended treatment on certain dates,
without being asked to offer an opinion regarding the patient's diagnosis or functional status.

If a therapist is asked by one of his or her patients to testify as an
expert witness, he or she should advise the patient that assuming a
dual role is likely both to destroy the effectiveness of the treatment
and to impair the value of any testimony. The therapist should recommend that the patient hire another mental health professional for
forensic evaluation and testimony. Many trial attorneys have difficulty understanding this issue. They are accustomed to calling treating orthopedists to testify in accident cases and fail to understand
that the psychotherapist-patient relationship involves another type of
process. Some attorneys are inclined to believe that a judge or jury
will more readily perceive a treating therapist to be believable than a
forensic expert. These attorneys argue that a forensic psychiatrist will
be criticized as being a "hired gun." In reality, judges and juries are
much more concerned about whether an expert appears to be a
knowledgeable and coherent person than about whether that profes-

sional has been hired as an independent evaluator.

It is important for the therapist who faces this situation to inform the patient of the risks involved. Patients and their attorneys are often unaware of the enduring nature of transference relationships. The special emotional bond between patient and psychotherapist provides an easy opening for the opposing counsel to prove that a powerful bias contaminates expert testimony offered by a treating clinician:

> Ms. Raven (opposing counsel): Dr. Selig, is it fair to say that over the period of time you have treated Mrs. Trane, you have developed considerable understanding and empathy for her problems?.
>
> Dr. Selig: Yes, certainly, I mean I certainly hope so.
>
> Ms. Raven: And does that mean that it would upset you if she became upset?
>
> Dr. Selig: Er, yes, of course.
>
> Ms. Raven: So shouldn't we assume that you would be upset to see her lose her case?
>
> Dr. Selig: Yes.
>
> Ms. Raven: How much does Mrs. Trane owe you, Doctor?
>
> Dr. Selig: Er . . . about $3,500 for her last 5 months of treatment sessions. Of course this doesn't include the $1,000 I will be charging her to testify today.
>
> Ms. Raven: As I understand it from what you have said here today, Doctor, she owes you a lot of money, you might not get paid for your testimony, and you are concerned that she will be upset if the jury doesn't accept her testimony. You have a lot riding on this case, don't you? This can't help but influence how you feel, can it?
>
> Dr. Selig: That's not how it really is, I'm just trying to tell it how I see it.
>
> Ms. Raven: I'm not implying that you are lying to us, Doctor, it's just that what you have told us here today might certainly have been influenced by your obvious conflict of interest in this matter. You have testified that you would not want to upset your patient. On top of that, she hasn't paid her bill in 5 months, and you haven't even been paid to testify. So if things don't turn out the way she hopes, she will probably be very

upset, and you might never see the $4,500 she owes you. As a psychiatrist, don't you agree that conflicts like that can color a person's attitude and opinion?

Dr. Selig: No! Er, why, yes, of course, but not in this case.

The therapist in this situation is in a double bind. If the patient loses her legal case, she might blame him for the outcome. If she wins, she might view him as a magic figure who has won her a pot of gold. Hearing the therapist testify about her in either a favorable or an unfavorable way might be a traumatic experience for the patient, as would seeing the therapist shamed in a devastating cross-examination. Forensic psychiatrists are required to interview other informants if possible, and this can be very intrusive and damaging to the therapeutic relationship. In any event, there is a high likelihood of irreparable damage to the treatment. It would have been better to have referred the patient to a forensic expert.

When patients insist that a treating therapist testify as an expert on their behalf and there is no way of persuading them to hire another professional to handle the forensic testimony, effective treatment has probably come to an end. The therapist in such a situation should arrange for a transfer of care. As part of the informed consent process, the therapist could tell the patient:

Clinical experience has shown that when a psychotherapist is called to testify by a patient as an expert witness, it is likely to cause irreparable damage to the treatment because it will interfere with our original goal, which was limited solely to helping you to get better. Testifying as an expert will mean that I will have to talk about you with your lawyer and other persons involved in your case. This will interfere with the previously private nature of our work together. I will have to get up in front of a courtroom of people and be asked many questions. I will have to answer them to the best of my knowledge, and some of the answers might be upsetting for you. It will change the whole nature of how we have been working together. It is also very likely to affect my objectivity as your therapist. Compounding things is the fact that this will all be happening at a stressful time during which you might need my therapeutic help the most. You are asking me to do something that

I do not think is good for you. As a therapist I cannot in good conscience do something that I believe would be bad for you. If you insist on calling me to testify in your case, I will have to refer you to the following colleague [give a specific name] for continuation of your care. I realize that seeing a new therapist can be disruptive, but that would at least enable you to continue with someone who will have a chance of providing proper care.

An effort should be made to explain the conflict of interest to the patient as part of informed consent. The discussion should be handled sensitively but firmly, with time given to allow the patient to work it through, if possible. In most cases, if the therapist stands firm, both patient and lawyer will agree to call another clinician as an expert. It may turn out that both patient and attorney were trying to exploit the therapist by intimidating him or her into becoming a low-cost witness. It may be necessary to obtain legal counsel in this type of situation if the therapist feels that he or she is being forced to do something that is against the patient's clinical interests. Therapists finding themselves under pressure to testify for an active treatment case should be aware of the American Academy of Psychiatry and the Law's (1987) *Ethical Guidelines for the Practice of Forensic Psychiatry* (Section IV) in this regard:

> A treating psychiatrist should generally avoid agreeing to be an expert witness or to perform an evaluation of [his or her] patient for legal purposes because a forensic evaluation usually requires that other people be interviewed and testimony may adversely affect the therapeutic relationship.

Contraindicated Treatment Arrangements

Prescribing controlled dangerous substances for oneself or one's family members. Prescribing such drugs for self or family is a very hazardous practice that may feed into a specific substance abuse syndrome. This practice is likely to be harmful to the "patient's" health, and may expose the therapist to legal sanctions (Winchell 1992).

Recommended Ways of Dealing
With Dual-Agency Violations

Covert signs of dual-agency violations. Therapy initiated under a dual-agency arrangement might proceed quite smoothly for an extended period of time. Like a time bomb, the explosion may be delayed. If patient A has referred patient B, one or both of them may be having dreams about being killed by a sibling; of Mother Hubbard in a shoe with too many children; or of an airline ticket agent who can't give out the correct scheduling information because he or she is overwhelmed with a glut of passengers. Patient A may take a turn for the worse, and this will upset patient B. Patient A may become romantically involved with patient B or with B's sibling. A and B may go into business together. All of a sudden, the seemingly trivial aspect of their connection has changed, and the therapist may find himself or herself preoccupied with keeping things separate. It becomes difficult for the therapist to conduct his or her therapeutic intervention with patient A without worrying about its effects on patient B.

Reparative responses. The vignette about Dr. Helms, Mr. Gordon, and Mr. Irving illustrates one way that a therapist might deal with such a problem in its early stages. Should a therapist find himself or herself in this predicament in its later stages, it is probably best to obtain consultation, depending on each patients' specific problems. The therapist might consider outlining the difficulty with one or both patients and going over the options according to the principle of informed consent (see Chapter 8). If the situation has not yet led to acting-out behavior, it may be possible to salvage both treatments. However, it may be necessary to refer both patients to different therapists if one or both are impulsive individuals and/or have "thin" ego boundaries.

CHAPTER 8

Respecting the Patient's Autonomy: Maintaining a Position of Neutrality

Whatever crushes individuality is despotism, by whatever name it may be called.

John Stuart Mill, *On Liberty* (1859)

Guiding Principles Regarding the Therapist's Respect for the Patient's Autonomy

Respect for patients' autonomy is one of the basic principles of medical ethics (Dickstein et al. 1991). It is best achieved when clinicians adhere to the principle of *neutrality*. In psychoanalytic technique, neutrality refers to the avoidance of taking sides in a patient's intrapsychic conflicts. This concept can be generalized to all psychotherapeutic modalities. In the most basic terms, neutrality means that therapists should avoid intrusive interference in their patient's personal life (R. I. Simon 1992a). Encouraging patients' autonomy entails maintaining a sense of separateness by avoiding physical and extratherapeutic social contact.

Neutrality may also refer to the idea of avoiding any misuse of patients' trust and dependency as a way of exerting power over them.

145

According to van Mens-Verhulst (1991), the issue of power in relationships can become quite problematic. Some clinicians strive for
"full equality," while others attempt to structure the relationship in a
more authoritarian way. Van Mens-Verhulst (1991) favored a model
that accounted for the fluidity of actual relationships. Employing this
paradigm requires being aware of the complex sharing and shifting of
power within the patient-therapist dyad. Patients and their therapists
have different sets of responsibility and power. As Peterson (1992)
has emphasized, therapists who deny any power differential are at
greater risk to commit boundary violations.

Dyer (1988) emphasized that clinicians need to be aware of the
conflict between the patient's desire for autonomy and his or her need
for dependency. Therapists can best resolve this dilemma by structuring the treatment to help the patient achieve as much independence
as possible. This process entails paying close attention to the patient's
unconscious as well as conscious communications. For example, a psychotic patient who begs to be sent home from the hospital prematurely may be testing whether the therapist is fully committed to a
treatment process that is likely to be stormy and arduous.

Adhering to the principle of patient autonomy does not mean
that therapists should abdicate their role of providing information and
guidance. Studies of medical populations (Ende et al. 1989) indicate
that most patients prefer that their physicians take the more dominant
role in treatment decisions. This model has been characterized as "pa-
ternalism with permission." Ende et al. (1990) found that physicians
in the patient role endorsed a similar pattern of response, although at
a less frequent rate than did nonphysician patients.

In practical terms, therapeutic interventions should be used
solely for a patient's health, safety, and well-being—not to pressure
the patient to adopt the therapist's value system and goals or to
provide the therapist with personal gratification. Encouraging the
patient's sense of autonomy is inherently ego strengthening. By maintaining a neutral position, the therapist conveys the following message to the patient:

> Your body, your mind, and your life belong to you. They are not for
> me to direct or take over. My role as your therapist is to help you

increase your understanding of yourself and your problems so that
you can deal with them better.

Appelbaum et al. (1987) emphasized that promoting autonomy
does not mean telling patients that they can do whatever they want.
Living in an organized society requires certain restrictions on personal autonomy, most notably when one individual's pursuit of gratification interferes with another's rights. As a result, therapists might
find themselves obligated to interfere with the autonomy of patients
who engage in dangerous behavior. For example, a therapist should
not stand idly by while a patient is imminently suicidal or homicidal.
Similarly, if a patient is actively abusive of another person (including
the therapist), intervention might be legally required. This does not
contradict the principle of autonomy; rather, it reinforces the idea
that freedom within a civilized group is a privilege predicated on
mutual respect for one another's personal space.

Indicated Ways of Encouraging Autonomy

Obtaining the patient's informed consent. Obtaining informed
consent involves educating the patient about the potential risks and
benefits of any treatment procedure. Guidelines for informed consent
regarding psychotherapy are not as firmly established as those
employed for prescribing psychotropic medication or using electro-
convulsive therapy (ECT). Nevertheless, discussing a proposed psychotherapy treatment plan is often the first opportunity for the
therapist to foster a patient's autonomy. The very act of offering a set
of choices and alternatives conveys the idea that the therapist believes it important for the patient to exert a key role in making
decisions about his or her own life.

Appelbaum et al. (1987) argued that the principle of autonomy
forms the core of informed consent for treatment. Basically stated,
informed consent refers to the right of any patient to make his or her
own decision about whether to enter treatment based on accurate
information regarding what type of treatment it will be and what risks
are involved. Lidz et al. (1984) reviewed the issue of informed con-

sent in psychiatry from a clinical, legal, and ethical point of view. These authors employed a disclosure model that fit both legal and ethical requirements, and attempted to determine its impact on patient care. Lidz and colleagues found that mental health care professionals in both outpatient and inpatient settings did not adhere very well to the model, and that the quality of patient care did not appear to be particularly correlated with efforts at fostering informed consent. Nevertheless, they argued for continued attention to this issue from the ethical viewpoint of encouraging patients' autonomy.

Like any intrusive procedure, psychotherapy has its hazards. It might be emotionally painful, regressive, expensive, or prolonged. According to Barnum (1992), informed consent involves a process of helping the patient to decide how to proceed with treatment recommendations. Three major questions are addressed:

1. What does the treatment entail?
2. What are the expected benefits and risks?
3. What are the viable alternatives to initiating treatment with the evaluating therapist? No treatment at all? A different treatment method? Would the same method with a different therapist be a better choice?

When the patient is a minor, these issues should be reviewed with the parents. Barnum emphasized that in order to be truly "informed," the consent decision must be *knowledgeable, voluntary,* and *competently made.* In work with children, Daws (1986) advocated looking at informed consent as an ongoing process that involves discussion and consensus building with the patient and his or her parents.

Despite the fact that many states require informed consent for treatment of any kind (psychiatric or otherwise), practitioners are usually afforded a "therapist privilege" (Lidz et al. 1984) that allows clinical judgment to be exercised in decisions about whether certain warnings might be damaging to a patient's well-being.

Informed consent for psychotherapy per se is a topic that is controversial and requires more study. Most therapists give a brief description of their proposed treatment plan. They let their patients know about the potential benefits without providing many details about risks or alternatives, often because they are concerned that too much information will confuse or frighten an individual who is already experiencing considerable distress. Such a patient may not be in a mood to listen to a long-winded, intellectual presentation about the risk-benefit ratio of a treatment plan. If the patient agrees to the therapist's proposed therapeutic regimen and evidences a sense of relief or a gesture of hopefulness, those indications are usually interpreted as consent enough. On the other hand, a more detailed, formal, and organized outline of the advantages and disadvantages of a specific treatment plan may impart a strengthening boundary message to the patient:

> This is your therapy; you play a vital role; there are alternatives from which you may choose.

Such a message can facilitate a more effective treatment process, in a fashion similar to that of Orne and Wender's (1968) role-induction interview for dynamically oriented psychotherapy. These authors noted that patients who were informed about the nature of psychotherapy beforehand were likely to have a better treatment outcome. The information Orne and Wender gave to patients as part of "anticipatory socialization" for therapy included the following:

1. The therapist informs the patient that direct advice is unlikely to be very helpful. Giving advice would encourage the unrealistic idea that the therapist knows "what is best" for the patient, when in reality, the therapist's expertise is most suited to help *the patient* find the best solutions.
2. The therapist explains that part of his or her role is to help the patient be more "honest" with himself or herself by pointing out conflicting feelings.
3. The therapist apprises the patient about "unconscious" mentation by explaining that he or she might recall being angry at a certain person and not knowing why. This might be a result of the fact that the person shares certain characteristics with another individual who has hurt the patient in some way.

4. The therapist warns the patient that therapy might cause changes that could be upsetting either to the patient or to his or her significant others. The patient might feel like he or she is getting worse, when the discomfort may actually be a sign of improvement. At such times, there may be a temptation to miss appointments or avoid treatment.

5. Talking about negative or angry feelings with an authority figure might seem like something that would ordinarily get the patient into trouble. The therapist encourages expression of such matters by letting the patient know that in the psychotherapy setting, it is important to tell the therapist about such thoughts and emotions, no matter how trivial or rude they might seem.

Much of the effectiveness of "anticipatory socialization" might come from helping patients to overcome their feelings of embarrassment in communicating with clinicians. Patients' shame in this regard probably derives from the perceived inequality of power in dependent relationships, intimidation, and fears of appearing foolish. Greenfield et al. (1985) demonstrated the importance of this aspect of health care in a randomized study of ulcer patients. Just prior to a medical visit, patients in the experimental group were encouraged to use assertive rehearsal, active questioning, and negotiation regarding medical decisions with their treating physicians. On follow-up, the experimental group reported significantly lower scores of physical limitation and role limitation than the control group.

Directly encouraging patient autonomy as part of the therapeutic method. Virtually every psychotherapeutic modality encourages patients to employ their inner resources to assist in the treatment process. Patients may be quite inspired to discover that their *own* ideas, feelings, and efforts are treated with respect—a finding that often results in a new way of experiencing themselves and the world. For example, in psychoanalytically based therapies, patients find that their dreams and free associations enable them to fathom secrets about themselves that they never thought possible. In cognitive-behavior psychotherapies, patients learn that they are able to provide critical information and feedback about their own beliefs and anxieties that helps the therapist to refine the treatment plan. They are gratified to find that it is their own efforts at applying the cognitive-behavioral "homework" that enable them to master situations that would have previously overwhelmed them. In hypnotically assisted psychotherapy, patients find that it is their own capacity for imagery and inner creation that enables them to recapture disconnected memories, to increase their inner sense of regulation and control of distressing symptoms, or to change their perspective of a problematic situation.

The therapist's role in encouraging patients to experience the power and value inherent in their own internal resources is quite analogous to Winnicott's (1951/1958) descriptions of the "good enough" mother who can provide a relationship within which the developing child is able to "create" and delight in its own mental productions.

Taking responsibility for treatment emergencies. When patients signal by word or deed that they are imminently suicidal or are soon likely to cause bodily harm to another person, it is important that the therapist respond in a timely and appropriate manner. Often, continued therapeutic work is all that is needed. At other times, it may be necessary to hospitalize the patient or to enlist his or her family's aid in containing the destructive impulses.

Readers might think it contradictory for me to list this type of intervention under the heading of "indicated ways of promoting autonomy." This issue is a source of widespread confusion. Patients who have temporarily lost control of the ability to protect their own bodies—or to refrain from acting on impulses to violate the bodies of others—are in imminent danger of being hospitalized, incarcerated, or dead. Therapists treating such patients are in a position similar to that of a parent who must prevent a child from running out into the street, or of an anesthesiologist who must breathe for a patient during surgery. It is a position of great trust. This responsibility should never be misused, but there are times when a responsible clinician cannot avoid taking action. Although the therapist intervening in such emergencies is temporarily taking control of the patient's body and "freedom," it is possible for most patients to internalize this behavior as a way of learning to take care of themselves and to restrain their own impulses. In such instances, the therapist is actually promoting autonomy by *modeling* appropriate self-care and restraint (Bratter 1975).

If required to take drastic measures, therapists should explore the patient's feelings about the intrusive intervention in an empathic but nonapologetic way. When patients are angry and confused about the seeming contradiction between a therapist who encourages independence on one hand and sets limits on the other, it may be helpful to explain that there can be no autonomy without self-governance. The following vignette illustrates this principle:

> Mr. Keel had made several suicide attempts while on a psychiatric ward. When placed on one-to-one observation, he tried to sign out of the hospital. His therapist, Dr. Loomis, told him that he was arranging for certification and involuntary hospitalization. Mr. Keel became furious and yelled at Dr. Loomis: "You have no right to take over my life! You are acting just like my overprotective mother!"
>
> Dr. Loomis replied: "Your suicidal behavior is a signal to me that *you are not in control of your life.* That is the problem. I am interested in working with you to regain that control. We can talk about the *thoughts and feelings* connected with your self-destructive wishes, but your *behavior* is not something that I can sanction. As a therapist, I am obligated to help you promote your health and safety, not to sit around while you destroy yourself. I don't think I would be helping you to become an independent person if I didn't respond in this way."

Relatively Risky Ways of Dealing With the Issue of Autonomy

Advising patients to make major changes in their life situation that are not related to exigent decisions about health or safety.   Therapists are often tempted to give direct advice regarding patients' major life decisions. This is particularly true with patients who present with highly dysfunctional and unsatisfying relationships. Tampering with a family system that has evolved into a stable pattern over many years is probably more dangerous than legislative efforts to revise the federal tax code. Unless an imminent threat to bodily safety exists or criminal behavior is involved, therapists should be wary of advising patients to break off long-standing relationships with a spouse or other relative. Unless the therapist has a comprehensive understanding of the purpose behind the complex and sometimes bizarre patterns that have evolved, efforts to pressure a patient to change are likely to be destructive. In most cases, the patient will not be able to follow the therapist's advice and will become demoralized for "failing" to cooperate. In other cases where the patient succeeds in following the therapist's advice against his or her inner judgment, the results can be disastrous:

> Ms. Maynard was in awe of her therapist Dr. Nolan. She idealized him and felt that he was the most wise, intelligent, thoughtful, and caring person she had ever met. Dr. Nolan appreciated these compliments, and looked forward to his visits with her. He thought of her as his "favorite patient." She complained bitterly to him that she could not stand the fact that her husband "was totally insensitive and ungiving." Dr. Nolan encouraged her to leave him, telling her that she "deserved better" and that this would improve her self-esteem. She reluctantly followed his advice. A messy divorce ensued. Ms. Maynard lost custody of her 8-year-old son when Mr. Maynard was able to prove to the court that she became incoherent during bouts of heavy drinking. Dr. Nolan had been unaware of her drinking patterns because Ms. Maynard had minimized the problem. It later turned out that many of Ms. Maynard's accusations against her husband were based on cognitive distortions and projection.

Dr. Nolan became intoxicated with the way that Ms. Maynard worshipped him. He accepted her fantasies about his infallibility as if they were reality, instead of a reflection of her need to assuage her impaired self-esteem. In effect, he began to see her as if she were an extension of himself, and therefore under his control and direction. His needed her praise to protect him against his own feelings of fallibility. This need prevented him from discerning the clinically important information required to treat her disorder. He needed to control her, and to see her as better than she was, as a way of defending against his own hidden feelings of shame (see Chapter 3 and Figure 3–7).

Attempting to influence patients to accept one's personal beliefs that have nothing to do with health or safety. In our study, 7.8% of 532 psychiatric respondents acknowledged trying to influence patients to support a political cause or position in which they had a personal interest (Epstein et al. 1992). Factor analysis showed that endorsing this behavior correlated with psychiatrists' disclosing personal details about themselves to patients in order to impress them, and with their talking about their own personal problems with patients with the expectation of getting sympathy. Even if patients appear to agree with the values that the therapist is endorsing, they frequently experience this type of pressure as an intrusive misuse of the treatment relationship. Encountering such behavior may weaken the patient's ability to trust the therapist as an objective and unbiased professional. It tends to remind patients of previous relationships in which a position of trust was misused in the service of personal gain.

Having difficulty allowing patients to separate from treatment. Our survey also revealed that 34% of psychiatrists responding found it painfully difficult to agree to a patient's desire to cut down on the frequency of therapy or to work on termination (Epstein et al. 1992). Therapists are often reluctant to see patients leave, even when the need for therapy is diminishing. This disinclination may be related to issues such as the painful sense of losing someone familiar, fears of abandonment, a hidden sense of shame over feeling rejected, and anxiety about the loss of income. Envy of the patient's growth and differentiation is another factor that can interfere with a therapist's ability to handle termination (Whitman and Bloch 1990). The case of Dr. Delphi and Mr. Eller in Chapter 4 illustrates the way that a therapist's envy can interfere with an otherwise successful treatment.

A patient's wish to either dilute or interrupt treatment may be a form of resistance that requires the therapist's active intervention. The therapist's valid technical objections to the patient's decision may be overshadowed by his or her affective state. The patient may hear the therapist's pain and conflict and not his or her words. Therapists who are better able to sort out their own feelings about being abandoned are in a more advantageous position to help the patient in this regard (Buie 1982–1983).

Contraindicated Ways of Dealing With the Issue of Autonomy

Seeking gratification by exerting power over patients.   Psychotherapy can exert powerful changes. While it is healthy and reasonable for therapists to be gratified by the sense of mastery and accomplishment obtained from successful work, this gratification should be a serendipitous by-product of the psychotherapy, not its goal. There is a danger for many therapists to become intoxicated by the power and influence that they have over their patients. Such feelings may lead them to forget that the purpose of treatment is to enhance the *patient's* well-being, not their own sense of professional self-worth. Many patients are exquisitely sensitive to this issue, and experience it as a form of psychological death if they perceive that another person has obtained a sense of mastery as a result of a relationship with them. These are individuals who may improve through "spite" cures. Their symptomatic relief occurs only in a way that leaves the therapist feeling helpless and confused. This is one of the reasons that therapists should never base their professional or personal self-esteem on the outcome of a single case.

We found that 49.9% of psychiatrists responding to our survey acknowledged that they felt gratified by a sense of power when they were able to control a patient's activities through advice, medication, or behavioral restraint such as hospitalization or seclusion (Epstein et al. 1992). Factor analysis revealed that these respondents were more likely to prescribe medications, make diagnoses, or offer psychodynamic explanations to their own family members and social acquaintances. This finding suggests that the temptation to misuse powerful psychotherapeutic methods in a clinical setting is likely to be replicated by similar behavior in the therapist's personal relationships.

Using power as a means of revenge against patients.   Psychotherapy can be a humbling experience. Patients often frustrate our
best efforts. They may surprise us by acting out in ways that are
perceived as "ungrateful," outrageous, and exploitive. Therapists
whose self-esteem is overinvested in a specific patient's outcome are
at increased risk for being overwhelmed by shame when they feel
"defeated" by a patient. Encountering such an affront can lead to
conscious or unconscious efforts on the part of the therapist to seek
revenge as a way of warding off the mortification associated with
feeling powerless, exploited, or vulnerable. (See Chapter 3 for a discussion of the "attack other" defense against shame.)

Retaliatory behavior is contraindicated because it conveys the
following message to the patient:

> I cannot stand the injury you have inflicted upon my self-esteem.
> Therefore, I am going to try to tear you down just as I feel you have
> done to me.

Taking revenge sets an improper role model for dealing with shame.
Maladaptive regulation of shame predisposes to other types of boundary violations. For example, some therapists initiate sexual involvement with patients as a reaction to their sense of powerlessness at
being unable to "cure" them. Their effort at forcing a "love-cure" is a
way of defending against the humiliation of feeling powerless. The
aggressive nature of the "romantic" seduction contains a hidden element of hostility and vengefulness.

Recommended Ways of Dealing With Boundary Violations Pertaining to Autonomy

Covert signs of violations of autonomy.   Reactions to violations of
autonomy are extremely varied. For some patients, complaints about
domineering parents, spouses, and employers are an indirect way of
communicating that they perceive the therapist to be overly controlling. Their dreams might include images of being tied down or imprisoned, or of desperate efforts to escape from confinement. The

therapist may find himself or herself locked in a power struggle with a rebellious and angry patient. The patient may act out his or her feelings by coming late, missing appointments, or threatening to discontinue treatment. He or she may attempt to employ countercontrol against the therapist and/or other persons. Another common manifestation is a therapeutic impasse. The patient passively seeks the therapist's advice but fails to improve.

Reparative responses. Therapists must differentiate their irrational need to "own" a patient from the patient's need to reenact a battle for control. If a therapist believes he or she has made significant mistakes in being overly restrictive or possessive, acknowledging and discussing these errors with the patient can be very therapeutic. Such a response serves to place the ball back in the patient's court, thereby allowing the patient to "reown" his or her part in the problem. If the patient decides to drop out of treatment as a result of autonomy conflicts, something useful and therapeutic can be salvaged if the therapist is able to structure an orderly and respectful termination. For example, if the patient states:

> Go to hell! You are nothing but a dictator who wants to rule my life! I'm leaving!

the therapist might respond:

> OK, I understand how furious you are with me. I don't agree with your decision to fire me on the spot, but it is certainly your prerogative. Regardless of what you decide, I think it's advisable for us to have one or two more sessions to give you an opportunity to talk about your feelings about what has happened and to reach some closure on this.

This approach leaves the decision in the patient's hands, while at the same time emphasizing the message that autonomy can be maintained without one party's having to destroy the other.

CHAPTER 9

Monetary Compensation in Psychotherapy: Balancing the Therapist's Financial Needs Against Those of the Patient

Socrates: Please tell me; what about the doctor in the most exact sense of the word, . . . is he a moneymaker or one who serves the sick? I mean the real healer? . . . the art of healing seeks no advantage for the art of healing but for a body. . . . then is it not true that no doctor, so far as he is a doctor, seeks or commands the advantage of the doctor, but only the advantage of the patient? For we have agreed, haven't we, that a doctor in the exact sense is . . . not a moneymaker?

Plato, *The Republic* 340E–342E[*]

Hillel: If I am not for myself, who will be for me? And in as much as I am only for myself, what am I?

Mishnayoth Nezikin, Avoth 1, Mishnah 14[**]

[*] Rouse (tr.) 1956.

[**] Blackman (ed.) 1965.

Guiding Principles Regarding Fees and Compensation for Psychotherapy

Monetary transactions between patient and therapist probably account for more boundary violations than inappropriate sexual involvement. Geis et al. (1985b) reported that whereas psychiatrists constituted only 8% of the physicians in the federal Medicare/Medicaid programs between 1967 and 1982, they represented 18.4% of individuals excluded from the programs because of fraud or abuse. Overrepresentation of Medicaid billing abuses by psychiatrists may be related more to the fact that they bill predominantly by the amount of time they spend with their patients, making it easier to prove a case of fraud against them than against physician specialists who bill primarily by procedure (Geis et al. 1985a). In their survey study, Pope and Vetter (1992) found that 14% of the ethically troubling incidents reported by psychologists were related to payment sources and third-party impingement on the treatment method. In contrast, sexual issues accounted for only 4% of the incidents. While sexual feelings can be managed solely through verbal communication, in private practice at least, the transfer of money from patient to therapist is a necessary behavioral aspect of the treatment relationship.

Employing factor analysis in our survey of psychiatrists, we discovered that one group of items from the Exploitation Index appeared related to monetary issues (Epstein et al. 1992). Although the range of the endorsement rate for the four criterion items was relatively low (2.3%–7.4%), in the main, they represent serious ethical violations. The key items loading on what we called the "greediness" factor included using information from patients, such as business tips or political information, for personal gain; undertaking business deals with patients; recommending treatments or procedures that are not necessarily in the patient's best interests, but that may contribute to the therapist's direct or indirect financial gain; and accepting a medium of exchange other than money for services (e.g., work on office or home, trading of professional services).

Feelings about money are a rich source of symbolism. They occupy a major role in the primary process interchange between patient and therapist. Compulsive preoccupation with money is frequently employed by individuals with pathological narcissism to defend against their feelings of embarrassment (Krueger 1986; see also the discussion of the "avoidance" defense against shame in Chapter 3). Shengold (1982) described some of the anal-erotic mechanisms underlying the practice of withholding payment of the fee and the important symbolic connections it may have with a patient's childhood memories of being seduced, violated, or exploited. Tulipan (1986) stressed how important it is for each therapist to evolve a coherent method of dealing with fees that is compatible with his or her own psychological makeup and working style. Drellich (1991) observed that therapists with small private practices were likely to feel highly dependent economically on each patient. He cautioned that this dependence could lead to ambivalent feelings of hostility.

Welt and Herron (1990) presented an excellent review of the narcissistic issues that operate within therapists to plague them over the issue of money. A major obstacle to clear thinking in this regard centers around the conflict between a therapist's wish to be an altruistic healer and his or her need to earn a comfortable living. Ablow (1992) has framed this conflict in a most poignant way:

> I rent my soul . . . I still feel embarrassed when my patients mention clinic fees. No matter how much I care for a patient, the fact that dollars are the life blood of the relationship seems to color my concern as impure—a hint of the prostitute feigning romance. (Ablow 1992, p. 35)

A hidden sense of shame regarding one's own worth as a person and clinician can interfere with a therapist's ability to deal with many patients who are burdened with similar conflicts. Welt and Herron (1990) described two types of illusory thinking concerning fees that are commonly observed among therapists. The first group takes a relatively permissive approach to fee arrangements because of a wish to have their patients perceive them solely as caring healers rather than as "money-grubbers." These individuals appear to be at increased risk when dealing with exploitive patients (see the discussion of the "attack self" defense against shame in Chapter 3). They are stunned by a patient's ingratitude. Conversely, they tend to overvalue patients who are more compliant. The second group of therapists handle fee arrangements well enough, in an organized and structured way, but attempt to justify their strictness regarding payment as being only for the patient's benefit. These therapists are resistant to allowing patients to question their motives. Both groups tend to set an unrealistic role model in financial dealings with their patients.

On a primary process level of thinking, psychotherapy is often equated with the love and caregiving of early childhood. This type of love is experienced as "unconditional." Having to pay for "love" can stimulate a profound sense of feeling abased and unworthy. Feelings of embarrassment and humiliation that are perceived by children during toilet training are undoubtedly linked to the fact that excretory continence represents the first major "condition" that the parents have placed upon their child in return for social approval. The desire to hide and the associated sense of shame so often connected with toilet training often results from the feeling:

> You no longer accept me as me, just as I am . . . your perfect and lovable child! . . . Now I have to do my duty in order to have you love me.

The growth of managed care as a major factor in the third-party payment of psychotherapy has created considerable debate among mental health professionals. Some groups have welcomed this paradigm as an opportunity to provide efficient short-term therapy that entails less worry about hassling for fees. In this vein, Appelbaum (1992) maintained that an organizational model would shield therapists from having direct monetary involvement with patients. He reasoned that private practice places therapists in a situation that pits their own interests against those of their patients. Under the organizational model, therapists have less incentive to cling to patients who no longer need their care.

Arguing against this point of view, advocates of traditional fee for service complain that managed care and related payment systems tend to create havoc with patients who require more treatment than is provided under the third-party plan. This often occurs because either the patient or the therapist feels pressured to stop treatment before it is clinically wise to do so. Although most managed care contracts clearly state that the therapist maintains full responsibility for all clinical decisions, the fiscal intermediary wields considerable power in the treatment process, particularly if membership on a specific managed care panel provides a significant portion of the therapist's yearly income. The fear of being dropped from participation because of an adverse practice profile could easily distract a therapist who was trying to work with a patient suffering from unusually complicated clinical problems (see Chapter 7 discussion of problems involving dual agency and conflict of interest).

Feldman (1992) noted that when the managed care organization places a financial premium on quick turnover and new intakes, therapists may develop a bias against patients who require lengthier treatment. She outlined various ways that the treatment relationship might become distorted through triangulating alliances formed between the therapist, the patient, and the health care organization. Feldman (1992) also emphasized how the payment modality can affect the way therapists view their patients' defensiveness against cooperating with the treatment process. For example, under a fee-for-service arrangement, it is not unusual to interpret the patient's "flight into health" as a denial of illness. In contrast, patients treated in a managed care setting who are unable to focus on well-defined, short-term goals are likely to be considered "resistant."

More quantitative evidence is needed to establish whether any pertinent relationship exists between treatment outcome and payment modality. Recent work by Rogers et al. (1993) suggests that prepaid plans may be associated with increased impairment among certain patient populations. For example, these authors found that depressed patients treated by psychiatrists under a prepaid treatment plan tended to acquire new limitations in their social or physical functioning over a 2-year period. The aggregate effect size was significant and relatively large, estimated as being equivalent to one-half of patients in the sample developing a single new impairment during the follow-up period. In contrast, patients treated in a fee-for-service setting did not develop new limitations.

Work by Rubin et al. (1993) indicates a similar pattern with regard to patient satisfaction with care. These investigators administered rating scales to a large sample of medical outpatients. A significantly higher percentage of patients treated in a solo-practitioner, fee-for-service setting scored their care as excellent, compared with those treated by multispecialty groups or health management organizations (HMOs). Clinicians scoring in the lowest quintile of patient satisfaction were four times more likely to have their patients drop out of care during a 6-month follow-up period than were physicians in the highest quintile. Although patients of mental health clinicians were excluded from data analysis, the obvious relationship between patient satisfaction and proclivity to cooperate suggests that these findings might be generalizable to psychotherapy populations.

Wachtel and Stein (1993) propose that fee for time is the most cost-effective way to pay physicians for their services. They argue that a stated hourly rate for medical services will encourage increased patient participation in the treatment process, reduce micromanagement and administrative expenses by third-party payers, and diminish the tendency for physicians to use procedural gimmickry to hide the true price of their services. Although it has been under considerable assault in recent years, fee for time has long been the traditional method of payment in private psychotherapy practice. In light of the emphasis placed on capitation fees and the resource-based relative value scale (RBRVS), it is interesting to see the fee-for-time model reenter the arena as a credible way of addressing spiraling health care costs.

Regardless of their opinions about the way therapy is financed, it is important for therapists to monitor the way that their patients respond to potential abuses. Learning how to resolve conflicting interests is part of social cooperativeness and human maturation. It is probably counterproductive to avoid dealing with a patient's conflicts over payment; rather, an effort should be made to confront such conflicts through exploration and discussion. Despite the fact that many patients receiving free treatment appear to do just as well as those responsible for paying a fee (Welt and Herron 1990), there may be certain individuals whose problems with self-esteem, entitlement, and motivation are incompletely addressed in a situation where payment issues are totally removed. Similarly, therapists are human beings who have a legitimate desire to earn a living through their professional work. Subtle efforts to hide or evade this desire might be an indication that the therapist is burdened with hidden conflicts of shame and devaluation about wanting to be compensated. The same issue of hidden shame may result in a feeling of quivering rage toward "ungrateful" patients who fail to pay their bills.

It is in the patient's best interest to have an opportunity to work through the narcissistic injury that arises in connection with having to give something in return for what he or she gets. Such a process is most likely to occur with a therapist who can deal realistically with his or her own economic needs while at the same time tactfully and sensitively assisting the patient to understand the feelings and issues that are stirred up by having to pay for treatment.

The following basic message is conveyed by a coherent compensation arrangement:

> Financial compensation is the only thing that you (or the responsible third party) are obligated to give to me.

Although it is natural for a therapist to seek general gratification from the pursuit of an interesting profession, this is not a burden that should be placed on any one specific patient. Many patients feel reassured when they have a therapist who is able to realistically communicate that he or she is a flesh-and-blood person who has realistic expectations regarding payment. This is particularly true for patients who have been accustomed to symbiotic and "pseudomutual" involvement in previous relationships. These patients have become confused by inappropriate role-reversal and covert emotional demands placed upon them throughout their lives and may perceive a coherent fee arrangement as an organizing and boundary-defining experience. Although on a primary process level the therapy fee may represent a "fecal" gift, on a more realistic level it can symbolize differentiation and self-respect. Paying for one's obligations strengthens boundaries.

Indicated Forms of Compensation

Fee-for-service or third-party coverage. Many therapists insist that their patients take direct responsibility for the fee, and that any third-party carrier reimburse the patient. This method has the advantage of keeping all financial transactions within the therapeutic relationship. Any tendency that the patient may have to withhold or delay payment is more likely to be available for immediate and direct discussion in the treatment setting. Accepting third-party assignment, with or without the patient paying a coinsurance balance, can be a workable method, provided that some formal structure is built into the contractual arrangement. As an illustration, the therapist might properly agree to receive direct payment of the 80% payment allowed by the third-party carrier, provided it arrives within a reasonable period of time (e.g., 60 days after billing). The patient may be responsible for his or her 20% copayment within 15 days after billing as well as for guaranteeing payment of the third-party portion if it is delayed past 60 days.

Accepting total assignment of the fee allowable by the third party appears to work with most patients. The way current trends in third-party payment seem to be going, assignment may become the primary mode of payment. Nevertheless, this modality may be not be the ideal arrangement for patients who suffer from severe narcissistic pathology, a marked sense of entitlement, or a need for acting out vengeful fantasies against authority. A similar situation holds for adolescent patients and adults whose treatment is directly financed by their relatives. Therapists need to be alert to the tendency of these patients to use the treatment as an suctioning device by which to drain their relatives and/or third-party carriers. Such a strategy may be an important element in their master plan for revenge. This is particularly likely in cases where there is a devil-may-care sense on the patient's part as to whether he or she comes to the appointments or whether the treatment results in symptomatic improvement.

Conversely, when relatives are paying for the treatment, a very real threat exists that they will sabotage the treatment, particularly when the patient begins to make some genuine progress. It is important to insist on a very explicit agreement between the patient and the relatives regarding payment at the outset of treatment. If possible, adolescent and financially dependent adult patients should be billed directly so that they carry the responsibility for obtaining the monthly check for payment from the relatives and giving it to the therapist.

This arrangement tends to short-circuit any tendency in "pseudo-mutual" families to diffuse their respective functions and boundaries by employing a "rubber fence." It helps to clarify the important boundary-defining concept that treatment belongs to the *patient*, not the family. It also helps to define the fact that the family's commitment to pay for treatment is with the patient, *not with the therapist*.

Full-time salary. Therapists who work as fully salaried employees in a clinic or health maintenance organization are spared most of the problems of collecting fees from patients or their families. However, other monetary issues can arise. For example, a therapist who feels resentful toward his or her employer may foster a misalliance with the patient that is organized around that resentment. The therapist may avoid confronting a patient who has failed to pay the required fee to the clinic, or may subtly encourage acting out by deflecting the patient's transference anger toward the "money-grubbing" employer. Such behavior may represent a way of trying to maintain the image of an "altruistic" therapist who gives only "unconditional love."

Token fee or gratis treatment. Many therapists are required to treat patients for token fees as part of their supervised work during training. Established therapists often donate a portion of their time to treat indigent patients in clinics or in their private practice. This is usually quite beneficial for patients who might otherwise be denied access to a more intensive treatment modality. On the other hand, therapists must exercise considerable caution when it is necessary to drastically reduce or waive the fee for a patient who has suffered a sudden financial reversal. Some patients experience "charity" as humiliating, demeaning, and engulfing. When they are no longer giving something of substantive value in return for the therapy, they may feel they have "ceased to exist" and can become depressed or suicidal. Flexible arrangements such as fee abatements, token payments made at the time of each session, or reduction in frequency of visits will usually serve to avoid an adverse outcome.

Conversely, patients who have been treated gratis as part of the therapist's pro bono work should be given the opportunity to start paying some fee if their financial status substantially improves. Such patients may develop an iatrogenically induced sense of entitlement and will have a hard time adjusting to a subsequent therapist who expects a more conventional fee-for-service arrangement (Horner 1991).

Charge for missed appointments.   It is customary for therapists to bill patients for missed appointments, especially when there has been insufficient cancellation notice. Some clinicians employ the metaphor that the regular psychotherapy session is equivalent to the rental on an apartment or the tuition for a college course. The time slot belongs to the patient for as long as he or she is enrolled. The therapist cannot arbitrarily give the time to someone else. The patient is therefore responsible for payment of the fee regardless of the amount of notice given or the reason for the cancellation. This practice is often misunderstood by patients and by other types of health care practitioners who are not familiar with treating mental disorders. The basic premise that justifies billing for missed appointments is that the patient is leasing a portion of the therapist's time as part of an overall program of regular care.

It is not easy for the therapist to fill a time slot if a cancellation occurs within a short time period prior to a given visit. Most patients rarely miss appointments, and for them it never becomes an issue. Other patients who frequently miss appointments do so because of problems related to their psychiatric disturbance, an unusual job situation, a disruptive family situation, or physical health problems. Having a clear policy of billing for missed appointments protects the therapist from being victimized by the peremptory claims of a patient who states: "How can you charge me for missing? I couldn't help it!" Responsibility for paying for appointments is a major factor in reminding the patient of his or her "ownership" of the treatment. The therapist's duty is to show up regularly and punctually. The patient's obligation is to pay for the sessions, even when attendance is not possible. This kind of arrangement maintains the viability of the treatment and prevents the web of guesswork and mind reading that would result if the therapist tried to undertake the impossible burden of deciding which reasons for patient absences were acceptable and which were not.

It is proper for therapists to negotiate with their patients about a temporary leave from treatment for reasons such as vacations, maternity leave, elective surgery, or extended business trips. These absences should be planned well in advance to allow the therapist time to rearrange scheduling.

Most third-party carriers will not pay the charges for broken appointments and take the position that a submitted bill should indicate if a specific charge is being made for a missed session. While many clinicians reason that it is the patient's responsibility to provide this information to the third party, submission of Current Procedural Terminology (CPT) codes for missed visits may be construed by third-party carriers as fraudulent claims (R. I. Simon 1992b). To avoid this risk and to maintain clarity and honesty, it would be reasonable to make an explicit note of any missed sessions on the claim form or to provide a general statement that some of the charges might be for missed appointments. Other types of billing notations can also address the issue of missed appointments (R. I. Simon 1992b). The patient should be informed about this procedure and of the possibility that the carrier will not honor the charges for missed sessions.

Therapists should become aware of Medicare and Medicaid regulations regarding the circumstances under which it might be illegal for them to bill patients for missed appointments. The regulations can be complex and confusing and are subject to frequent changes. Medicaid regulations differ from state to state and may be quite restrictive. As an example, in Maryland, the code governing health care rendered to Medicaid patients clearly states:

> The provider may not bill the Department for ... (2) Broken or missed appointments (COMAR 10.09.02.07 Payment Procedures. J.)

Under current Medicare regulations as of May 1993, broken appointments fall under the category of procedures that are "not covered" (Medicare Medical Policy Bulletin No. Z-24, p. 1, June 17, 1991). According to Betsy A. Boswell, Supervisor, Beneficiary/Physicians Services, Pennsylvania BlueShield/Medicare (personal corre-

spondence, May 24, 1993, obtained under the Freedom of Information Act), Medicare regulations do not prohibit physicians from billing *patients* directly for missed appointments, as long as the amount
billed does not exceed the limiting charge allowed for the procedure
that would have taken place if the patient had attended. Even
though all physicians have been required to file Medicare charges for
their patients since September 1, 1990, Ms. Boswell noted that physicians need not submit charges for broken appointments to *Medicare*
unless the patient requests an official denial statement. Under Section 3043 of the Medicare Carrier's Manual (02–93), if the patient
desires a formal Medicare determination for a service that is not
covered, the physician must file the claim and is instructed to indicate on the form his or her belief that the service is noncovered and
is being submitted at the beneficiary's insistence. Ms. Boswell stated
that when a patient makes such a request, the physician should report
the procedure as a broken appointment under CPT–90899. Since
CPT–90899 (unlisted psychiatric service or procedure) is a nonspecific identifier, a notation should be included explaining that the
procedure is a broken appointment. This avoids any ambiguity or
misinterpretation about the nature of the charges. For the same reason, it might be best to use the CPT–90899 code and notation on
any bills sent directly to the *patient*.

Regardless of which third-party payer is involved, I think it a
reasonable corollary to the practice of billing for missed sessions for
therapists to take financial responsibility for their own scheduling
snafus. To illustrate:

A patient appears for her scheduled appointment and discovers
that her therapist is not present. She has taken 2 hours' leave from
her job to attend the visit. The therapist was delayed at the hospital because of a crisis on the ward and was unable to notify the
patient before she departed from work for the session.

Consistent with the principles of maintaining coherent boundaries, it would be useful to convey the idea to the patient that her
time is just as valuable as the therapist's. The therapist might compensate the patient for her lost time by offering a monetary credit on

the bill that could be used for a subsequent session. Although it might be reasonable for the therapist to explain why he or she missed the session, this should not be used to deny responsibility for compensating the patient for her inconvenience. The patient should not be burdened with deciding if the therapist had a "good reason" for missing the session, just as the therapist should not have to decide this for the patient. The embedded message contained in this practice is the idea that both therapist and patient are responsible for their own behavior, not each other's.

Relatively Risky Compensation Arrangements

Working at salary for an organization one perceives to be financially exploitive of its employees. Salaried therapists who receive a disproportionately low percentage of the income generated by their clinical efforts are likely to feel used by the management and to experience considerable anger. Patients seeking treatment in such a setting are at risk of being caught up in unconscious acting out and "enabling" with their therapist. The atmosphere in institutions that exploit their employees may closely resemble the internal dynamics of the dysfunctional families in which many patients were raised. Such a treatment environment can be toxic and antitherapeutic.

Accepting gifts of small monetary value. A gift from a patient, no matter how inexpensive, is a form of communication in action rather than in speech. A gift always has a symbolic meaning (Talan 1989). By accepting it, the therapist is allowing a short circuit in the verbal mode of communication and a breach in the therapeutic "frame." Gifts, like idolatry, often represent a "living sacrifice"—a form of compensation that is outside of the contractual agreement. The patient may be trying to bribe the therapist so as to avoid feelings of shame, guilt, or anger. Therapists usually fear refusing a gift out of concern that their refusal will humiliate the patient. This fear may have more to do with the *therapist's* feelings of shame than with the patient's. Tactfully exploring the thoughts and feelings behind the gift, explaining why gifts in general might be counterproductive for the therapy, and exploring the patient's feelings about the refusal can all be very useful. By encouraging the patient to explore any feelings of abasement and hurt connected with refusal of the gift, the therapist communicates the powerful message that *no feeling* is beyond exploration or containment within the treatment frame. Talan (1989) suggested that the therapist can address this issue in an empathic way by acknowledging that the patient could be finding it difficult to use words to convey his or her inner experiences at a given moment in time, and that the gift may be an effort to communicate "that which cannot be spoken." On the other hand, if the gift is accepted, the therapist may inadvertently signal to the patient:

> Some emotions [like shame] are beyond your [and my] capacity to talk about. There is no way of dealing with them directly. We have to cover them over.

Supervisory folklore has long advised therapists in training to accept gifts of small value from schizophrenic patients, particularly when they are paying virtually no fee. The reasoning is that such patients are already burdened with cognitive confusion and extremely low self-esteem. It is argued that they will experience an organizing sense of validation by being able to give some token of worth to the therapist. Similarly, R. I. Simon (1992b) believes that gifts of small value cause no harm, particularly when given at the termination of treatment. However, even with psychotic patients, if the therapy is of long duration and the gifts are repeated on a regular basis, the therapist should consider exploring the issue in terms of its function for the patient's self-esteem.

Bartering goods or services in return for psychotherapy.   Although barter might be a necessary form of trade at certain times, it is a risky form of payment for psychotherapy. Payment in chickens is not well standardized. Money is a measurable and fungible commodity that has a fixed value at any given point in time. Barter introduces the idea that one party might "best" the other in the deal. For example, a therapist might agree to accept a struggling artist's paintings as payment in lieu of a fee. Such an arrangement carries a high risk that one of the parties will end up feeling exploited. The patient might later perceive that the therapist has gotten a "steal" if his or her work begins to sell at premium prices. On the other hand, the patient might unconsciously spoil the quality of his or her work out of resentment.

In other cases, therapists have been known to permit their patients to perform skilled services such as accounting, secretarial work, home construction, and legal services in return for treatment. This situation usually involves an increasingly personal involvement between patient and therapist. R. I. Simon (1989) cautioned that this type of arrangement often occurs during the "prodromal" phase leading up to sexual involvement with patients.

Referring patients for treatments or procedures in which one has a financial interest. Referring a patient for tests, procedures, or treatments that are based primarily on the therapist's proprietary interest in a lab, hospital, diagnostic center, medical device manufacturer, or drug company exposes the patient to the risk of a biased recommendation. Patients often sense they are being "milked" into giving additional and uncontracted remuneration. This practice has led to intense public discussion and a call for regulation by statute (American Medical Association Council on Ethical and Judicial Affairs 1992; Crane 1992). The American Medical Association Council on Ethical and Judicial Affairs (1992) believes that abuses around self-referral undermine physicians' professional commitment.

Mitchell and Scott (1992) found that over 40% of physicians in Florida had investments in health care businesses (other than direct care practices) to which they referred patients. Crane (1992) emphasized that physician self-referral may interfere with the ability of other practitioners who do not own a secondary facility to compete on a level playing field based strictly on cost, quality, and convenience. He argued that this practice has created a negative image for medicine, has eroded the public's trust, and has not provided much in the way of benefit for patients.

Financial conflict of interest is a complex issue, and there are many arguments on both sides of the question. Therapists wishing to protect the treatment boundaries and minimize any risk to their patients should make full disclosure about any financial interest they have in a specialized treatment or diagnostic modality. The therapist should also provide information on alternative sources for the procedure, including a brief review of relative costs and a risk-benefit analysis. Even if no practical alternatives to the procedure exist, the therapist should carefully explain the situation to the patient and inquire about any negative reactions to the proprietary interest.

Neglecting lapses in a patient's adherence to payment as contracted. A patient's failure to meet the terms of the fee arrangement constitutes a breach in the therapeutic boundary. It is important that the therapist confront and explore the behavior, even if the lapse seems trivial (e.g., a payment shortfall of $1.00 in a bill of $400). Therapists are often reluctant to focus on such minor infractions because they do not wish to be perceived as carping or excessively concerned with money. Some patients will intuitively play on this ambivalence, and may vociferously criticize the therapist once he or she finally screws up the courage to discuss the problem. There is a good chance that the patient is covering up feelings of guilt or shame and projecting them onto the therapist. Because such conflicts may play a key role in the patient's psychotherapy, a full recovery may not be possible without tactful confrontation.

Contraindicated Compensation Arrangements

Engaging in fraudulent financial practices. Fraudulent practices include deliberate deception about time billed, false marketing claims, deliberately inflating reported costs to justify higher fees with regulating agencies, and billing for services that were never scheduled with the patient and therefore never rendered. Fraudulent billing should be clearly distinguished from the legitimate practice of billing for missed appointments, in which the patient was provided with a reserved time slot that he or she never used. Therapists who exploit their patients and third-party payers by engaging in fraud are often attempting to compensate for their own conflicts over weakness and vulnerability. Bergler (1959/1970) observed that compulsive fraud is rooted in efforts to repair narcissistic wounds. Embezzlers, frauds, and impostors tend to act out a pattern of unconscious revenge in a futile effort to repair lesions in their self-esteem.

The therapist who is overconcerned with money or who feels a sense of "entitlement" because he or she is so talented and "special" may be harboring large-scale defenses against feelings of shame and inadequacy. He or she exports these unbearable affects by projecting them onto the patient. When the "victim" is the third-party carrier, the therapist teaches the patient a corrupt and maladaptive way of soothing narcissistic wounds.

Splitting fees. This practice involves a "kickback" for a referral. It is a fraudulent practice because the referral to the other clinician is based solely on financial motivation. It is deceptive because the patient is led to believe that the referral is a reasoned professional decision based on his or her clinical needs.

Accepting gifts of substantial value. Large gifts cause a big-time corruption of the purpose of treatment. They may be in the form of expensive items, cash, or bequests. These gifts are usually offered at the end of a reasonably successful treatment by a "grateful" patient (see the case of Dr. Delphi and Mr. Eller, in Chapter 4, for a vignette concerning this issue). The therapist who accepts such gifts is grasping defeat from the jaws of victory. Rothstein (1991) presented a case of an older man who offered to leave him a bequest for $250,000. Instead of accepting this seductive offer, he encouraged the patient to explore the possible meanings of his proposal. This annoyed the patient, but he was able to uncover fantasies of achieving eternal care by supporting the therapist's work with handicapped children. It turned out that the patient's prior therapist had sent him a letter a number of years after termination soliciting funds for a psychiatric foundation.

In this type of situation, the patient is acting out a wish to "purchase" the therapist as a way to prove that the latter really a corrupt person. By taking the "bait," the therapist probably undoes the treatment. The offer of a large gift presents the therapist with an opportunity to show his or her "true" stuff. It provides a good chance to explore the meaning of relationships and to solidify the gains in treatment.

Colluding with patients to deceive a third party.   This practice involves entering into a fraudulent misalliance with the patient. Secretly waiving the patient's copayment has been construed as fraud by some insurance companies (R. I. Simon 1992b).

Using "insider" information.   Therapists have been subjected to criminal and civil sanctions for trading on secret or proprietary information that has been revealed in the course of a patient's psychotherapy session (R. I. Simon 1992b).

Recommended Ways of Dealing With Boundary Violations Pertaining to Compensation

Covert signs of violations.   Patients who feel cheated by their therapists may report dreams of being overcharged for admission to a theater, being "fleeced," or being involved with gangsters. Conversely, patients who are late in paying their bills may dream about hoarding stockpiles of cash or shoplifting. If the therapist has accepted a gift, the patient will often report dreams that can give a clue as to the gift's symbolic meaning. Deviant fee arrangements often lead both therapist and patient to project their conflicts onto each other. For example, a patient who tends to act fraudulently with other persons may attempt to get the therapist into legal trouble by tricking him or her into deceiving the insurance company. The following case history illustrates some of the difficulties that arise when a therapist permits the formation of a deviant treatment frame. In the initial portion of the vignette, the first therapist unquestioningly accepted the patient's hidden frame. The subsequent therapist was able to search out the meaning of the deviant frame and was then able to establish an effective and workable treatment.

> Ms. Oakes was a 35-year-old woman suffering from anxiety, mild depression, and low self-esteem. She sought therapy from Dr. Percy.

She had recently ended a relationship with a man with whom she had lived for 5 years. She was mortified that this man had pressured her into "lending" him money from her limited savings to support his compulsive gambling habits. He never repaid the loan.

Ms. Oakes told Dr. Percy that she was "poor" and could not afford his usual fee of $100 per session. He agreed to lower his fee to $80. Ms. Oakes then asked that he bill her insurance company $100 per session, since they would pay up to 50% of $100, or $50. She would pay him the extra $30, to make up the difference between $50 and $80. If he recorded the expected fee of $80 on the insurance form as his actual charge, the company would only pay 50% of $80, or $40. She told him she had "terrible cash flow problems" and could not afford the extra $10 copayment. Dr. Percy agreed that he would record the charge on the insurance form as $100, even though they both knew she would never be responsible for more than $80.

After several months of treatment consisting of once-weekly psychotherapy sessions and benzodiazepines, Ms. Oakes' anxiety had intensified. She began to miss appointments. She complained that no man could ever find her attractive. Despite Dr. Percy's efforts to reassure her about her attractiveness, Ms. Oakes abruptly terminated treatment without paying her last bill or submitting the final insurance form.

Several months later, she sought help from Dr. Quincy because her symptoms had intensified. She was very impressed with Dr. Quincy's sensitive comments at the conclusion of their initial interview. However, she became defensive and embarrassed when Dr. Quincy told her that she could not go along with the idea of maintaining two sets of fees, one for the patient, and one for the insurance company. Ms. Oakes became enraged when she was informed that Dr. Quincy would also feel obligated to make notations on billing statements identifying any missed appointments. Dr. Quincy tactfully endeavored to explain why it would be illegal and counterproductive for Ms. Oakes' treatment and personally risky for herself as a professional if she failed to adhere to this format. Nevertheless, Ms. Oakes bitterly complained that she could not understand this position: "Your rigidity is unfairly depriving me of my first real opportunity to get treatment from someone who seems to understand me!" She cried bitterly, and pleaded with Dr. Quincy that she could not afford to see her without this special arrangement.

Dr. Quincy was distressed and quite puzzled. She searched for clues as to the origin of this affective storm. She suspected a projective mechanism and asked the patient if anyone had ever attempted to deceive *her* in her life (as she realized that Ms. Oakes was begging her to do with the insurance company). Ms. Oakes looked at the therapist in amazement and tearfully recounted how she had been cheated out of her inheritance by her maternal aunt. Her mother had died when she was 10 years old. Her aunt, who became her guardian, had connived to embezzle a major portion of her mother's estate. The aunt later lost the money in a series of speculative investments but had managed to sequester the remaining portion for herself, which she never shared with the patient. This had been the start of great financial hardship for the rest of the family. Dr. Quincy suggested to Ms. Oakes that she might be attempting to reenact this terrible sense of betrayal in the treatment setting. The double-fee arrangement might be an unconscious effort to test the doctor out to see if *she*—like her aunt and former boyfriend—was also a corrupt and reckless person. Ms. Oakes listened very thoughtfully. She confirmed Dr. Quincy's tentative explanation with further historical information. She told the therapist that she might be willing to dip into her savings to pay the coinsurance on the fee because she felt for the first time that she had found a trustworthy person who might be able to help her.

Reparative responses.   If a therapist realizes that he or she has violated a boundary by accepting a gift, it is appropriate to try to correct the situation by explaining the nature of the problems this action has created for treatment and returning the gift. If the therapist discovers that the method of remuneration has been corrupt, it makes sense to restructure the arrangement and take responsibility for any financial loss. If the therapist misses a session without notice, causing the patient lost wages and lost time, it is reasonable to credit the patient for an extra session in compensation.

When the patient is trying to exploit the therapist in regard to the fee, the therapist should confront the issue. A continuation of the previous vignette serves as an illustration:

Several months later, after the treatment had become established, Ms. Oakes was 5 days late in paying her bill. She became enraged when Dr. Quincy asked for payment. Ms. Oakes stormed at her: "You have so much more than me, how come you can't make any allowance for my impoverished condition?" Dr. Quincy replied: "Like you, I have financial needs. I also have rules and agreements that I have to follow. If I allow you to take advantage of me like your aunt and boyfriend have done with you, I am not only letting myself be hurt, but also setting a very poor example to you about how to deal with other people who might try to exploit you in the future." Although she continued to complain bitterly about the therapist's "money-grubbing" attitude, Ms. Oakes paid her bill and continued her therapy. She gradually became more effective in her relationships at work and socially. She became involved with a man who was both financially stable and considerate of her needs.

C H A P T E R   1 0

Confidentiality

Who is the bearer of gossip? One who carries things that have been spoken and goes from here to there saying, "So-and-so said this" or "This is what I have I heard about so-and-so." Even if what he says is true, behold this person destroys the whole world.

Moses Maimonides (1135–1204 A.D.),
Mishneh Torah, Hilchot De'ot 7[*]

El pez muere por la boca. [The fish dies because he opens his mouth.]

Spanish proverb

Guiding Principles
Regarding Confidentiality

A patient owns his or her thoughts, emotions, and secrets. This is the basic meaning of patient privilege. The privilege belongs to the *patient*, not the therapist. R. I. Simon (1992b) defined the rule of confidentiality as the "ethical duty of the psychiatrist not to disclose information obtained in the course of evaluating or treating the patient to any other individual or party without the express permission of the patient. . . . The consent, however, must be given competently, knowingly, and voluntarily" (pp. 52, 63).

---

[*] 1944 (ann. Birnbaum).

Aside from certain exceptions governed by societal and legal mandates, any communication between patient and therapist should be seen as taking place solely for the purpose of treatment. Such communications must therefore be kept secret. Respect for the obligation of confidentiality transcends the therapist's judgment about whether or not the unauthorized release will be harmful to the patient. It is not the therapist's right to decide that an inappropriate disclosure is harmless just because he or she doesn't think the patient will suffer any adverse consequences. When patients discover that information has been released without authorization, they often feel as if a piece of themselves has been misappropriated. By maintaining a patient's confidence, a therapist transmits a defining behavioral message that is trust-enhancing and ego strengthening:

> Your secrets and your communications belong to you (the patient), not to me (the therapist). Only *you* have a right to reveal them.

Indicated Ways of Keeping Confidentiality

Insisting on proper authorization from the patient before releasing information. Unless authorized by the patient, no information should be released to a third party, not even the fact that the therapist knows who the patient is. It is easy for therapists or their office staff to reveal damaging information unintentionally. For example, during Richard Nixon's successful bid for the presidency, a reporter telephoned the office of Nixon's previous medical psychotherapist and asked about the details of the former vice president's treatment. The doctor's secretary told the caller that she could not release any information on Mr. Nixon because all information on their patients was confidential. However, in so doing, she revealed that he had in fact been a patient. This "noninformation" became the source for the next day's banner headlines. The story illustrates the need for therapists and their staffs to have a prepared "canned" response when confronted with unauthorized requests. For example:

Caller: This is the XYZ insurance company; we need to verify that you are treating Mr. John Zilch.

A stock response would be:

Therapist: I don't release information about *any* patient unless I receive a properly executed authorization.
Caller: So you are telling me that all you need from me is to send an authorization from *your patient* Mr. Zilch?
Therapist: No. I am telling you about the laws and ethics of confidentiality. It is improper for any health professional to discuss any information about a patient, even whether the professional knows that patient, without valid authorization.

In responding to requests for information from insurance companies and other third-party payers, it is important to obtain the patient's authorization. For ongoing cases, it may be useful to encourage the patient's prior review of all outgoing correspondence and to ask him or her to take direct responsibility for dropping such information in the mail. This approach tends to foster the patient's "ownership" of his or her communications within the treatment.

Giving appropriate feedback to a follow-up source.   For new patients, it is usually appropriate for the therapist to thank the referring clinician and to provide a follow-up call or letter regarding the patient's diagnosis and proposed treatment plan. This information should be geared to the referring practitioner's "need to know" and should not involve gossip about clinically irrelevant information. Ongoing discussions with the referring clinician may be necessary if he or she is to play a continuing role in the patient's care. For example, an internist might need to monitor potential medical complications from psychotropic medications. When ongoing collaboration with another clinician is anticipated, the general nature of the disclosure should be discussed with the patient beforehand.

In situations where one psychotherapist refers a patient to another psychotherapist, continuing follow-up discussions after the initial period of transfer of care usually constitute a breach of confidentiality unless the patient has authorized such additional discussions. The referring therapist has no lingering connection to the case once the transfer of care has been completed. His or her interest in the outcome may be legitimate, but that information does not "belong" to either of the therapists; it belongs to the patient. It is reasonable to discuss the case with a former therapist if such communication is part of a supervisory arrangement. Sometimes the two therapists are expected to consult with each other because each are working with different members of the same family. In such cases there should be a clear understanding on the part of *all* patients concerned as to the nature of the discussions and the constraints involved.

Informing the patient of any anticipated dangers to confidentiality. As part of the principle of informed consent, the therapist should warn the patient about possible limitations to confidentiality in those situations where it appears likely to be a significant issue. This knowledge will enable the patient to have an informed choice in weighing the risk-benefit ratio of whether to reveal or not reveal certain information. Patients raising their mental health as an issue in the course of a lawsuit should be warned that all revelations to the therapist are potentially discoverable by the opposing litigants. Discovery may involve the right of the other side to take testimony from the therapist in a deposition and/or to obtain photocopies of all written records. Although this situation might significantly impede the patient's ability to speak freely in the therapy, it need not prevent some useful treatment from occurring.

   Other exceptions to confidentiality vary by jurisdiction, and include the mandated reporting of child abuse, abuse of the elderly, patients suffering from mental or physical conditions that impair safe use of a motor vehicle, patients who have made serious threats to harm others, and previous therapists who have sexually exploited the patient (see Table 1–1). Leong et al. (1992) have reviewed some of the dilemmas involved with these issues. In Massachusetts, psychotherapists who are psychologists and social workers are required by statute at the initiation of treatment to warn patients about the various limitations to their privilege unless the clinician documents that such disclosure would cause a serious deterioration in the patient's mental state (Beck 1992; Mass 1988 Chapter 112:129A Rec 251

CMR 3.07). For example, under this statute, the therapist must inform the new patient that a judge will have the discretion to order release of the psychotherapy records of divorcing spouses in child custody cases if examining them is deemed in the best interests of the minor children. According to Beck (1992), a similar statute in Texas also requires such reporting but without the clinical discretion allowed in Massachusetts.

While it is important for therapists to be aware of these issues, it is both impractical and countertherapeutic to try to provide advance warning to every patient about all possible dangers to confidentiality. Legally mandated transfer of information without the patient's consent does not necessarily destroy the treatment, and may even at times be therapeutic. For example, some patients will not be able to stop abusing their children until their own therapist reports them to the authorities. Treatment does not necessarily end at this point. Even if the patient suffers legal sanctions as a result, this action may actually strengthen the treatment alliance. If the therapist has forthrightly explained his or her legal obligations to the patient and the reasons for the disclosure, the patient may respect the therapist for being true to his or her beliefs in following the law. He or she may also be able to identify with and admire a therapist who refuses to collude with destructive behavior by keeping an abusive secret.

Discussing treatment issues with parents of child and preadolescent patients. It is customary to conduct ongoing and fairly open discussions of treatment issues with the parents of young children who are in psychotherapy. Children ages 12 or younger expect the therapist to speak with parents as part of their care. Nevertheless, treatment may be impeded if the child is fearful that the therapist will reveal certain issues to the parent. It is important to listen for the child's cues in this regard (Daws 1986).

Including members of family therapy or group therapy in the contract for confidentiality. All participants in conjoint family and group psychotherapy become privy to sensitive and personal revelations. Therapists customarily orient new group therapy patients by explaining the need for maintaining confidentiality (Yalom 1970). In the District of Columbia, mental health professionals are required by law to give a written statement to prospective members of therapy groups informing them that there is a prohibition against revealing confidential material and delineating the legal penalties of noncompliance (District of Columbia Mental Health Information Act of 1978, D.C. Law 2–136; Kearney 1984). Before patients are actually allowed to enter the group, they must sign a statement indicating that they understand the law and are willing to abide by it.

Davis and Meara (1982) reviewed the issue of confidentiality in group therapy. Members requiring external support or seeking self-enhancement were more likely to disclose group secrets. These authors also found that adherence to confidentiality was positively correlated with group cohesiveness. R. I. Simon (1992b) stressed that it was important for therapists to be aware of the legal pitfalls regarding confidentiality under the aegis of group therapy, even when conducted outside of those few jurisdictions that provide statutory protection. He reasoned that it is the therapist's responsibility to monitor group members' ability to agree to keep all information within the confines of the therapeutic situation. It is conceivable that a therapist could be held responsible for any damages resulting from poor clinical judgment in this regard. For example, it would not be a good idea to allow a poorly controlled manic patient into a group where other members were in the habit of discussing potentially damaging information. The manic patient might not be able to adhere to limits on secrecy.

Obtaining supervision and consultation.   Supervision is essential in the training of all psychotherapists. After the completion of formal training, many therapists continue ongoing supervision with a respected colleague or obtain ad hoc consultations when they are troubled by a difficult case. Ongoing peer study groups are also a very effective way of obtaining ongoing professional advice. Supervisors are obligated to follow the rules of confidentiality. Any breach violates the trust both of the therapist who sought consultation and of the patient who relied on the therapist's judgment. Therapists seeking individual or peer supervision should select individuals who are known to be reliable in this regard.

Relatively Risky Forms of Managing Confidentiality

Engaging in planned or unplanned communications with members of the patient's family. Discussing a patient's case with the patient's relatives requires considerable care. Family members of an individual psychotherapy patient will often pressure the therapist to discuss the patient's care with them. This is most likely to occur when the patient is an adolescent or young adult who is dependent on the family, has poor ego functioning, is regressed, or is displaying alarming symptomatic behavior.

Although it may be reasonable to release information in an emergency situation, unauthorized discussion of a patient's case with his or her relatives can be quite damaging to some patients. Such an action can exacerbate a crisis, precipitate sudden termination of treatment, or provoke serious symptomatic regression. Many patients process *ex parte* discussions with family members as a sign of the therapist's fundamental lack of respect for their personal existence or worth. The basis of the patient-therapist relationship is communication. If this communication is treated as the therapist's property, it is as if the patient's ownership of his or her thoughts has been completely discounted.

Demands for release of information often come from family members who have difficulty accepting the patient's autonomy. In many cases, this aspect of the relatives' behavior plays an important role in the patient's psychopathology. Similar problems arise during inpatient treatment (Uchill 1978–1979), where many individuals are privy to the chart and there is a greater pressure on the therapist to have communication with family members.

Communicating with family members may be essential in certain situations mandated by clinical and legal conditions. It is best if the clinician is able to anticipate the possibility of such interactions with third parties and to discuss this with the patient in advance. If emergency conversations with the family are necessary, an effort should be made to have the patient participate.

Adolescent patients being treated in an individual paradigm

should be informed at the outset that the therapist believes it best to keep confidentiality. The therapist should make it clear that certain actions on the teenager's part might necessitate communication with his or her parents, such as dangerous behavior (the therapist might be legally required to notify them) or provocativeness (the parents might be pressured into making disruptive demands on the therapist or pull the patient out of treatment). It is important to see the parents at the beginning of treatment to obtain collateral history and to establish the guidelines for confidentiality. Gabel et al. (1988) recommend that the therapist inquire about any family secrets and about whether the parents have any objections to their disclosure to the child. Parents have legal rights and responsibilities and should be included in the process of informed consent regarding the risk-benefit ratio of psychotropic medications and procedures. On the other hand, all parties should be informed of the probable adverse effects to the treatment if ongoing transfer of information with the parents occurs during psychotherapy. In those cases where the patient's clinical status requires continuing collateral involvement of parents, the ramifications and limitations of this involvement should be discussed beforehand. Even in such circumstances, the therapist should monitor the patient's reactions to this transfer of information. The same issues apply to treatment of adults whose disturbances are severe enough to warrant family concern and intervention. It is probably best to include the patient in all conversations with family members that may be required, both at the initial collateral interviews and subsequently.

Discussing patients with one's colleagues, family members, or friends. It is fairly common to overhear therapists discussing their treatment cases in social situations. Sensational and potentially damaging material is revealed in front of nontherapists who may be present. Other therapists regularly discuss their cases with spouses and family members who are not trained mental health professionals. We found that 67.9% of psychiatrists in our survey study disclosed sensational aspects of a patient's life to other persons, even if they believed they were protecting the patient's identity (Epstein et al. 1992). R. I. Simon (1992b) observed that therapists with "loose lips" unveil the secret information with which they have been entrusted as an exhibitionistic display of power. Disclosures of this kind are used as a way of impressing others with one's special role as a "guardian of secrets." For some therapists, divulging such information is a way of showing off that they are privileged to treat "important people." As tempting as it may be, discussing confidential information is a dangerous practice from a number of standpoints. Often, the patient can be identified even if his or her name is withheld. A piece of the public trust in psychotherapy is eroded every time one of our colleagues talks casually about patients under his or her care. Unauthorized revelation of information can cause significant damage to patients' personal relationships, reputations, job status, and the outcome of litigation. In one case of which I am aware, a psychiatrist started speaking about his patient at a social gathering without mentioning the patient's name. One of the guests replied, "Oh, I know who you are talking about!" She accurately identified the patient, and proceeded to tell about her relationship with him.

It is a breach of confidentiality to discuss details of a specific psychotherapy case with family members who are not also mental health professionals. Such conversations violate the spouse's or relative's boundaries by placing them in a role reversal. The family members are usually expected to admire, console, or advise the therapist without having the benefit of either the training or the mantle of professional authority that would enable them to coherently carry out such a task. True love and "total openness" with one's spouse does not justify revealing professional secrets. Any self-respecting spy knows that telling one's spouse a state secret places him or her in jeopardy. An analogous situation holds for therapists. Relatives should not be burdened with the task of maintaining confidentiality when they have neither the training nor the knowledge to understand the full implications of being privy to such information. A careless slip by a spouse could lead to injury for the patient and a lawsuit for the offending therapist.

Releasing information about deceased patients.   Patients do not lose their right to confidentiality when they die. This principle applies to famous personages as well. Authorization by heirs does not justify disclosure if release of the information has not been explicitly authorized by the decedent prior to death. As R. I. Simon (1992b) indicated, the decedent may have died wishing to keep certain sensitive information from his or her children, and has a right to take these secrets to the grave. The privilege belongs to the patient. R. L. Goldstein (1992) recently reviewed the issues involved in a case in which a therapist disclosed the records of a deceased famous patient without having received her explicit approval.

Presenting clinical material at a conference or for publication. Advances in any scientifically based discipline require that there be collegial sharing of clinical information and experience. Society's need for well-trained health professionals justifies this process. R. L. Goldstein (1992)˙ reviewed the arguments for balancing this need against patients' right to confidentiality. The dilemma is best handled by careful efforts to disguise the identity of patients whose cases are discussed in any publication. In some instances, a case cannot be camouflaged without vitiating its clinical value; perhaps such material should not be written up. Arguments regarding the important scientific aspects of a case may conceal the therapist's desire for self-aggrandizement.

Clifft (1986) provided an excellent set of guidelines for disguising clinical material in situations where therapists believe that a case contains sufficient value to justify its preparation for publication. She pointed out that it is risky for authors to assume that patients will not see their own case report just because it was published in an obscure journal. She emphasized the importance of disguising the presentation to the point that even the patient himself or herself will be uncertain as to the identity of the person involved. R. I. Simon (1992b) advised that the disguise should be sufficiently complete to prevent a close friend of the patient from recognizing his or her identity.

Contraindicated Forms of Release

Releasing information to third parties without authorization, legal authority, or other mitigating reason. In the absence of an authorized release, requests for information from third parties should be refused. A breach of this rule is likely to seriously interfere with the patient's ability to trust the therapist. At times such an impropriety can lead to injurious consequences that neither the therapist nor the patient could have anticipated. Offhand remarks to a colleague who is treating a relative of a patient may trigger problems between the patient and his or her family member. For example, R. L. Goldstein (1989) reported a case in which a patient sued his psychiatrist for releasing information to his wife. He claimed that the disclosure led to the breakup of his marriage. The court agreed with the patient's claim, stating that in the absence of an "overriding concern," the risk of unauthorized disclosure to a spouse would deter people from seeking the help they needed. In some cases, release of information becomes a discoverable "leak" that opens the door for testimony in a lawsuit, which could lead to the patient's suffering monetary loss in litigation, loss of a job, or loss of a strategic advantage in a business deal (R. L. Goldstein 1989).

Third parties frequently make unauthorized requests. Such requests are often couched in ways calculated to elicit shame in the therapist. The embedded message is "How can you be such an unfeeling and uncooperative person as to refuse a simple request?" Because this induced feeling of shame appears to center around the high value that most therapists place on being helpful and facilitative, it is important that therapists be prepared for the demeaning intonation and subtle pressure that frequently accompany unauthorized requests. Many people, even trained therapists, simply fail to understand the high risks involved. Some third parties, such as relatives of the patient, attorneys, journalists, and other health care professionals, are quite aware of the laws regarding confidentiality, but use guile to intimidate or trick the therapist into revealing forbidden information. Therapists must understand their obligations in this regard, regardless of whether anyone else does.

Patients should be included in the decision both of *whether* to release and of *what* to release. One effective practice is to discuss the risk-benefit issues of disclosure with the patient and to show him or her any written reports that are to be released. Some therapists give such reports to the patient in an unsealed envelope so that he or she has the physical responsibility of reading the material and putting it in the mail.

A therapist who receives a subpoena to release records and/or to appear for a deposition regarding a patient should not assume that there is a legal requirement for immediate disclosure. He or she should inform the patient *before* taking any action. If the patient refuses to release the information, his or her attorney may successfully quash the subpoena, depending on the legal issues involved. In situations where patients are unable to provide for their own legal protection, it may be necessary for the therapist to consult his or her own attorney for legal assistance in blocking the subpoena.

An exception to the requirement for confidentiality arises when the therapist is required to take emergency action. For example, he or she might need to seek civil commitment for an uncooperative patient who is imminently dangerous to self or others. In some states, *Tarasoff* laws may require that a therapist warn third parties if he or she has reason to believe that the patient is likely to inflict violent harm upon them. Therapists are advised to become familiarized with local law in this regard, both because it varies widely according to jurisdiction and because the information disclosed should not exceed the amount required to warn the person(s) in danger. According to R. I. Simon (1992b, p. 308), the original *Tarasoff* ruling stated:

> The warning to a victim should be done in such a way as to preserve confidentiality consonant with the prevention of threatened danger.

R. I. Simon (1992b, pp. 297–344, especially pp. 307–310) has provided a cogent review of the complex subject of *Tarasoff*-type rulings and the way they affect confidentiality.

Releasing information to third parties even when authorized, if the potential for adverse consequences is suspected.   It follows from the doctrine of informed consent that the therapist has a responsibility to warn a patient if clinical experience indicates that disclosure of information is likely to be damaging. The therapist should avoid colluding with the patient's plan for disclosure under these circumstances. Rather, he or she should discuss the hazards and explore the patient's underlying motivation for taking such a risk. A request for release to third parties not directly involved in the current care of the patient may be an invitation to help the patient act out unconscious self-destructive fantasies. To illustrate:

> Mr. Gevalter was a successful scriptwriter whose career was forcefully promoted by his ambitious mother. He called up his former therapist, Dr. Heil, and told him that he had arranged an interview with a TV talk show host and wanted his doctor to publicly discuss the content of his psychotherapy on a nationally televised program. Mr. Gevalter told Dr. Heil that he had written about his treatment in his new autobiographical novel entitled "My Therapist, My Healer." Advance reviews were quite promising, and this was a great opportunity to promote the book. He told Dr. Heil that he had asked his attorney to prepare a signed release authorizing any disclosure Dr. Heil deemed appropriate. This would be enclosed with a check for $7,500 to cover the doctor's expenses and to allow him to share some of his newfound success. Mr. Gevalter told him: "Everything is all ready to go, if you are agreeable."

Should the therapist honor Mr. Gevalter's request, just because the patient has given written authorization? A terminated treatment, no matter how successful, is never immune to retroactive sabotage. The patient is probably making an unconscious test of the therapist's integrity—asking, in effect, "Are you more interested in promoting your own fame and feathering your own nest (like my mother) than you are in taking care of me? Are you ready to sell yourself out to me, just as I did for her?" In this example, the therapist is presented with a golden opportunity to help his former patient and to protect the past therapeutic gains. Dr. Heil could suggest that the patient come in for a follow-up visit so that he could make an appropriate interpretation:

> Dr. Heil: "I think we should look at the meaning of your request. Were I to accept your tempting offer, I would be allowing you to purchase me, just as you felt your mother did with you. Could this be a way you are testing me to find out if I am a real doctor? You

may be trying to find out if I am a true healer interested primarily in your well-being, rather than an exploiter who just wants to feather my own nest."

Further caution is required in dealing with signed releases. With current patients, signed releases are usually not a problem—the therapist will have already been apprised about the need for the specific transfer of information, and any doubts about the release can be discussed with the patient before action is taken. However, if a therapist receives a release from a third party purportedly signed by a *former* patient, it would be prudent to contact that patient to verify the signature. This extra bit of concern is particularly important if there is any uncertainty as to the identity of the third party requesting information, or if the patient's records contain potentially stigmatizing information. If authentication by telephone is possible, the therapist is also afforded an opportunity to caution the patient about any special risks that might be involved in releasing the information.

Recommended Ways of Dealing With Boundary Violations Pertaining to Confidentiality

Covert signs of violations of confidentiality. Patients who sense a breach in confidentiality may report dreams with images of intrusion and exposure. Such dreams may include scenes of the psychotherapy being conducted in an airport waiting room; of coming to a session without clothes on; of being dissected by the therapist in front of a group of medical students; or of watching the therapist host a radio talk show. The patient's associations may center on an acquaintance who "can't keep his or her mouth shut" or on children who are "blabbermouths." Some patients might identify with the therapist's porous confidentiality boundaries by imitating his or her behavior— for example, by making self-destructive revelations of their own secrets. Others will clam up and stop reporting dreams. Their verbal productions become more stilted and superficial.

Reparative responses. Most breaches of confidentiality consist of seemingly harmless lapses that the patient never knows about. There is no direct damage because the third party either has no connection with the patient or forgets about the revelation. Therapists who are aware that they behave in this way should endeavor to restrain themselves. Like driving while intoxicated, the fact that an action doesn't seem to do any harm doesn't mean it isn't dangerous. Repetition increases risk. Therapists who find themselves repeatedly making exhibitionistic remarks about their patients during social gatherings should ask themselves if they are employing an "avoidance" defense against shame (see Chapter 3).

Another issue arises when a patient learns that the therapist has spoken to his or her relative or insurance carrier without previous authorization and discussion. Unless the communication has caused obvious trouble, most patients will not voice objections to the therapist's behavior but will evidence one or more covert signs of the type mentioned above. If the therapist detects a reaction of this kind, he or she should discuss it with the patient in terms of its relationship with the previous breach in confidentiality. Such a discussion strengthens boundaries and serves as a way of defining the importance of the patient's privilege and of his or her ownership of the therapeutic communications.

CHAPTER 11

Maintaining Anonymity

One confidence deserves another, and anyone who demands intimacy from someone else must be prepared to give it in return. . . . But this technique achieves nothing towards the uncovering of what is unconscious to the patient . . . he would like to reverse the situation and finds the analysis of the doctor more interesting than his own. . . . The resolution of the transference, too—one of the main tasks of the treatment—is made more difficult by an intimate attitude on the doctor's part, so that any gain there may be at the beginning is more than outweighed at the end. . . . The doctor should be opaque to his patients and, like a mirror, should show them nothing but what is shown to him.

Sigmund Freud,
"Recommendations to Physicians
Practicing Psychoanalysis" (1912)

Guiding Principles Regarding Personal Disclosure

Freud's (1912/1958) original advice regarding anonymity has been applied in various forms to psychoanalysis and other psychodynamic therapies that work directly with transference phenomena. It remains valid in psychoanalytic work (Siegel 1985–1986) and can be generalized in some ways to other forms of psychotherapy.

Since the therapist is not a disembodied spirit communicating from out of the void directly into the patient's ear, it is impossible for him or her to be perfectly "opaque." Opacity is not an end in itself. The purpose for restraining personal revelation is to maintain a single-minded and strictly professional focus on the patient's problems. It is a method to avoid being sidetracked. Flooding patients with gratuitous information serves to rivet attention on the therapist's personal life and detracts from the purpose of the treatment.

Therapists who are able to refrain from revealing unnecessary personal information communicate the following message to their patients:

> This treatment is for you, not for me. I am not going to burden you with my personal needs and life interests, because you are not here to take care of me. I am going to resist any temptation to let my own worries sidetrack us from working on your problems.

Indicated Forms of Self-Disclosure

Giving the patient information about one's training and treatment methods.   As discussed in Chapter 8, the principle of autonomy dictates that patients should be given the opportunity to exercise informed consent regarding the proposed treatment plan. Patients are entitled to know that the therapist is properly trained and to have a chance to decide whether his or her therapeutic orientation is consistent with their own life goals.

Discussing reality factors that directly impact on the patient's decision to enter or continue treatment.   Therapists should inform patients when their practice plans or health status are likely to have a significant impact on treatment decisions. For example, if a therapist is planning to retire in 2 years, new patients who require long-term therapy should be informed of the likelihood of having to find a new therapist before their treatment can be completed. If a therapist has a serious illness that might cause a temporary or permanent interruption of treatment, the patient should be given enough information to allow him or her to deal with the realistic impact on the treatment and to provide for transfer of care if necessary.

Even a dying therapist has a responsibility to maintain a professional posture with his or her patients. For example, a therapist with terminal cancer should inform patients that he or she has a fatal disease that is probably incurable. A brief statement of the diagnosis and prognosis is reasonable to help orient the patient to reality and probability of outcome. It gives the patient an opportunity to grieve the loss and to enlist the therapist's help in saying good-bye. It affords the possibility of achieving some closure. Excessive detail about the nature of the therapist's disease and treatment probably places an unnecessary burden on the patient. Discussion of anatomical pathology and procedural techniques can traumatize some patients with frightening images that may be internalized in unpredictable ways. Alexander et al. (1989) reported on the death of their colleague, an analytically oriented clinician, of terminal cancer. This clinician sought peer support to help her work through the process of informing her patients about her diagnosis and prognosis. This helped her to maintain a professional stance with her patients and assisted her patients in working through their feelings of disruption and loss.

Discussing reality factors that may be needed to "contain" a disturbed patient's anxious fantasies. During the exigencies of treating severely disturbed patients, it may become necessary for the therapist to provide the patient with a "reality check" to help a patient who is having difficulty distinguishing fantasy from actuality—or self from other. For example, acutely suicidal patients may experience a sudden reduction in the intensity of their self-destructive impulses if the therapist is able to express his or her personal sense of caring and concern. A depressed woman with mood-congruent delusions might believe that she has caused her therapist to become contaminated and diseased. It is appropriate for that therapist to reassure the patient about his or her own health status. A man with borderline personality disorder who has developed an intense, erotized transference toward his female therapist might proclaim that he hopes that her husband will die of natural causes so that he can marry her. It might be useful for the therapist to inform the patient that she wouldn't marry him even if he were the last remaining man on earth. Paranoid patients often develop terrifying anxiety as a result of their delusions that the therapist is involved in a plot against them. They may experience considerable relief if the therapist lets them know, in no uncertain terms, that such behavior is not consistent with his or her own ethical standards.

The important element in each of these cases is that the therapist limits the disclosure to specific information required to help the patient to cope with distressing beliefs or impulses.

Relatively Risky Forms of Self-Disclosure

Informing patients about minor details of one's personal life, particularly if the purpose is to impress patients, manipulate their behavior, or gain sympathy. Personal disclosure by therapists is fairly common. Borys and Pope (1989) found that 38.9% of psychiatrists, psychologists, and social workers acknowledged in a survey that they disclosed details of current personal stresses to a patient. In our survey, 16.7% of the responding psychiatrists made personal disclosures about themselves in order to impress their patients (Epstein et al. 1992). We also observed that 7.8% talked about their own personal problems with patients with the expectation of receiving sympathy. As previously mentioned in Chapter 8, factor analysis showed that both items regarding self-disclosure factored together with the tendency to pressure patients to go along with the psychiatrist's political and personal interests.

Inappropriate personal disclosure may endanger the integrity of the treatment because it is a signal to the patient that the therapist is interested in reversing roles (see Chapter 4), is departing from the strictly professional stance as a caregiver, or has problems with self-restraint.

Contraindicated Forms of Self-Disclosure

Making repeated disclosures about one's family relationships, marital problems, personal worries, and psychological conflicts. Experience has shown that unrestrained and repeated self-disclosure about intimate life problems is often employed by erotic practitioners. It is a common precursor to their sexual involvement with patients

(Brodsky 1989; Schoener and Gonsiorek 1990; R. I. Simon 1992a). Even when no sexual behavior takes place, some patients may respond to such disclosures by becoming suicidal because they experience them as a sign of the therapist's exploitiveness and lack of integrity (J. Simon 1989). Extensive personal disclosure may be a sign of a severe impairment in the therapist's ability to understand and maintain the professional role.

Recommended Ways of Dealing With Boundary Violations Pertaining to Anonymity

Covert signs of violations of anonymity. Patients may have very ambivalent feelings about a therapist's personal disclosure. On one hand, they may become irritated because they feel that the therapist is "cutting into their time." Conversely, they might feel pleasurably impressed with a sense of the therapist's friendliness, and they are being made to feel important. On an unconscious level, patients may experience their therapists' revelations as a seduction or an attempt to impose their own values. They may have dreams about policemen who reveal information to the criminals; about navigational markers that have been placed in the wrong location; or about watching the therapist's spouse having sex with the therapist. They may make offhand remarks about friends who are like "shoemakers who don't stick to their last." Accommodating patients may react by reversing roles and attempting to become the therapist's healer. Impulsive patients, especially those with porous ego boundaries, may act out damaging sexual and aggressive scenarios. These behaviors can sometimes be traced to elaborate derivatives of the seemingly innocent personal details the therapist has revealed in previous sessions.

Siegel (1985–1986) presented two case histories illustrating ways that patients in psychoanalytically oriented therapy may react unconsciously to a therapist's disclosure:

> The therapist announced that she was planning to go on a summer vacation. When the patient asked if she would be available for a

session or phone consultation in case of need, the therapist stated that she was "planning to go to abroad with her family and therefore would not be available" to the patient. Although the patient appeared to accept this response, he noted that he could not remember the dream he had the previous night. He started to talk about his brother's female boss, whom he disliked because she "runs off at the mouth." He remarked that he felt that this woman behaved inappropriately because she acted like she had a personal relationship with him that she did not have and that he did not want. "She did not know where to stop, and he did not like that in a woman . . . she had gone too far . . . her behavior was flirtatious." The patient then went on to talk about a man whom he had been trying to get to help him with his taxes. He then added that the man was really strange and that he was no longer in the tax business. He was now making pornographic movies . . . he was probably starring in them, too.

Reparative responses. Although Siegel's case is drawn from a psychoanalytically oriented therapy, the issues it demonstrates can relate to other modalities as well. The material derived from the patient's primary process closely reflects his perception of the therapist as intrusive, inappropriate, seductive, and exhibitionistic. Monitoring these responses would give the therapist an opportunity to gain a better understanding of the way that the patient responds to breaches in the boundary. For example, he or she might assist the patient in seeing the connection between the disclosure and the feelings of role-reversal. Acknowledging the effect of the revelation increases the likelihood that the patient will be able to discuss other situations in which he or she had to worry about a caregiver's narcissistic sensitivities.

Therapists will often disclose personal information in response to a patient's direct questions because they are afraid the patient will feel humiliated and rejected if they fail to respond. This assumption may relate to the therapist's own defenses against similar feelings. Gabel et al. (1988) noted that child psychotherapists are often quite concerned about appearing unpaternal or unmaternal with their patients. In an effort to avoid antagonizing the patient, they will usually answer questions about their personal life without inquiring about the reason for the child's interest. They emphasized that such questions provide an opportunity to help focus the child on the importance of the child's own ideas and feelings in the therapy process.

It is possible to deal with offhand questions about the therapist's personal life in a tactful way if the therapist is able to resolve his or her own feelings about being in a situation similar to that of the patient. For example, if a new patient asks if the therapist is married or where he or she was born, it is important to provide a courteous, nonrejecting explanation of why this information is being withheld. If the therapist judges that the question is not a vital "reality check" that should be answered directly, he or she might say to the patient:

> "I'd like to hear about your interest in this and to know more about it and any other questions you have, but I prefer not to reveal information about my personal life to you. Doing so could alter my special professional role with you, which is for me to listen to your thoughts and feelings rather than for me to burden you with mine."

On a conscious level, at least, most patients will accept this as just another aspect of the therapist's professional demeanor. Some patients will feel rejected no matter how the matter is phrased, and it is important to follow up by asking how the patient feels about the therapist's refusal to answer the question. The emotional reactions are often unconscious. For example, any disclaimer by the patient notwithstanding, a rejected question may be perceived as a tyrannical prohibition against all questioning. It is important to anticipate this and to be able to listen for the patient's reactions. To extend the example:

> When asked about his reaction, the patient might say: "Oh, I understand, it's no problem, that's the way doctors work." He might then start talking about how oppressed he feels by his supervisor, who is like his father who had to be obeyed "unquestioningly." The therapist is then in a position to remark: "So maybe the fact that I refused to answer your question makes you feel like I'm an autocrat who can't be challenged in any way. It's really OK with me for you to ask me questions. It's just that sometimes I have to handle them as if they were like any other thought that comes into your mind.

Some of them I can't answer because I have rules I have to follow, so that I can do my best job in my effort to assist you."

Abstinence and the Management of Erotic Feelings in Psychotherapy

For him [the analyst], it is an unavaoidable consequence of a medical situation, like the exposure of a patient's body or the imparting of a vital secret. It is therefore plain to him that he must not derive any personal advantage from it. The patient's willingness makes no difference; it merely throws the whole responsibility on the analyst himself. . . . It is rather, perhaps, a woman's subtle and aim-inhibited wishes which bring with them the danger of making a man forget his [psychotherapeutic] technique and his medical task for the sake of a fine experience. And yet it is quite out of the question for the analyst to give way. However highly he may prize love, he must prize even more highly the opportunity for helping his patient over a decisive stage in her life.

Sigmund Freud,
"Observations on Transference-Love:
Further Recommendations on the
Technique of Psychoanalysis" (1915)

Guiding Principles for Dealing With Sexual Feelings in Psychotherapy

Therapists should apply the principle of abstinence when it comes to dealing with the feelings of sexual excitement and arousal that they experience with patients. Freud (1919/1958, pp. 162–163) defined *abstinence*, in its broadest sense, as follows: Therapists shouldn't short-circuit the patient's urges by rushing to gratify them; patients are best served in therapy if they express their feelings through words, rather than action. This advice protects the patient from his or her own emotions and impulses as well as from those of the therapist. Therapists who adhere to this principle set a healthy role model for dealing with conflict. Four basic behavioral and verbal statements are thereby imparted to the patient:

1. "Your mind and body belong to you. No one [not even I, your therapist] is allowed to take liberties in this regard."
2. "The sole purpose of this treatment is to foster your health. Its purpose is not my gratification."
3. "There is an enormous difference between feelings and actions. It is possible to have strong desires and not act on them. There are other ways of handling such feelings without being swept away by them."
4. "Our relationship is solely for your treatment, and regardless of any emotions either of us might experience, it must never lead to a direct life involvement like that between friends, acquaintances, relatives, or romantic partners."

When coherently applied, these messages tend to encourage the patient's sense of self-respect and integrity. Although some patients may initially feel gratified by romantic involvement with their therapist (Apfel and Simon 1986), such involvement ultimately fosters dependency rather than individuality, impulsiveness rather than frustration tolerance, and feelings of being exploited rather than a lasting sense of accomplishment. With some patients, erotic involvement with the therapist even increases the risk of suicide (Pope and Bouhoutsos 1986).

The great majority of therapists report that they occasionally experience sexual feelings for patients. For example, Pope et al. (1986) found that 95% of male psychologists and 76% of female psychologists reported experiencing such attractions on at least one occasion. Despite the ubiquity of these feelings, many therapists are confused and troubled by them. Such difficulties may increase the risk for boundary violations.

Gabbard (1991) reviewed a number of characteristics that could serve to alert therapists that they are at increased risk for becoming sexually involved with a patient. A common theme pervading these issues is a marked tendency to confuse desire with behavior (see Table 12–1).

Whenever a close empathic connection arises between therapist and patient, it has the potential to stimulate sexual arousal in one or both parties. By carefully analyzing these feelings instead of acting on them, the therapist is likely to obtain useful information about the patient's projective identifications. On the other hand, the relatively high frequency of psychotherapist-patient sexual involvement suggests that dealing with issues of erotic feelings and sexuality can become problematic for a significant number of therapists. Studies of surveys conducted between 1973 and 1989 have revealed that from 0.5% to 13.7% of therapists acknowledge engaging in sexual behavior with patients. A detailed breakdown from some of these studies is given in Table 12–2.

Schoener (1990) has provided the most comprehensive review to date of the survey literature on mental health professionals' acknowledged sexual contact with patients. A weighted average that I calcu-

Table 12–1.   Characteristics of therapists who are at increased risk for erotic involvement with patients

- The therapist confuses his or her own need to be loved as an indication that it is actually the patient who requires love.

- The therapist is burdened with the pervading fantasy that love cures all ills.

- The therapist's enthusiasm to help the patient is transformed into romantic behavior.

- The therapist-patient relationship develops toward a reenactment of the patient's incestuous history.

- The therapist has a proclivity to harbor resentment toward his or her former teachers or therapists, and acts out such feelings with rebellious and maverick-like disregard for the usual rules of abstinence and restraint with patients.

Source.   Adapted from Gabbard 1991, p. 655.

lated from Schoener's tables (excluding a very large national sample of nurses) revealed that 7.38% of male therapists and 2.29% of female therapists acknowledged having sexual contact with patients. These figures were derived from 10 studies involving a total of 5,816 respondents, broken down by gender. Because the studies had very divergent response rates and methodologies, the averages should be viewed as only crude approximations.

Survey data also indicate that even among those clinicians who deny sexual involvement with their patients, a high percentage have a rather fluid view of the physical boundaries with patients, and they have difficulty differentiating the specialized therapist-patient role

Table 12–2. Percentage of therapists acknowledging sexual involvement with patients on survey studies conducted between 1973 and 1989

Authors/Population studied	Percentage acknowledging involvement
Kardener et al. 1973	
Male psychiatrists	10.5
Perry 1976	
Female psychiatrists	0
Holroyd and Brodsky 1977	
Male psychologists during therapy	5.5
Female psychologists during therapy	0.6
Male psychologists after termination	2.6
Female psychologists after termination	0.3
Gartrell et al. 1986	
Male psychiatrists	7.1
Female therapists	3.1
Pope and Bouhoutsos 1986 (citing Forer 1980)	
Male psychologists	13.7
Borys and Pope 1989	
Male and female therapists[*] during treatment	0.5
Male and female therapists[*] after termination	3.9

[*]Study included psychiatrists, psychologists, and social workers.

from that of an ordinary social relationship. For example, Borys and Pope (1989) found that 29.9% of clinicians admitted becoming friends with a patient after termination; 10.3% invited patients to an office/clinic open house; 8.0% employed a patient; 7.2% invited patients to a personal party or social event; and 11.6% went out to eat with a patient after a session. Similarly, in our study, 18.8% of the psychiatrists we surveyed had pursued a posttermination relationship with a patient; 45.2% touched their patients (besides shaking hands); 30% felt gratified by a patient's seductiveness; 24.7% thought of a patient as possessing more gratifying qualities than their own spouse; and 33.2% took pleasure in romantic daydreams about a patient (Epstein et al. 1992).

Indicated Forms of Physical and Emotional Involvement

Shaking hands. A handshake is a generally accepted form of greeting and leave-taking in many cultures. Individuals raised in the United States will often extend a handshake at the first meeting with a therapist but not thereafter. In contrast, patients raised in European and Latin American societies frequently expect to shake hands at the beginning and end of each visit or, at the very least, before a vacation. Except for the initial meeting, it is my view that the therapist should not attempt to initiate a handshake with a patient. On the other hand, if a patient regularly offers to shake hands with the therapist, this in itself is unlikely to create much of a boundary problem if it remains within stereotyped cultural patterns. However, even when it is culturally expected, a handshake may cause difficulties for patients in intensive psychodynamic therapy and those with a poor conception of their spatial boundaries (Szekacs 1985). It may be useful in such cases to advise the patient against regular handshake except for the initial and final visits of treatment. The reason might be explained as follows:

> It's a nice and friendly custom for people to shake hands when they say hello or good-bye, but since our relationship involves a special

way of working together to help you with your problems, and since treatment works best if all of our communications are put into words, I advise against our shaking hands until your treatment is completed.

Patients who have been previously traumatized by exploitation or abuse can be very reassured by this attitude because it is a clear message that the therapist has thought this matter out beforehand and takes his or her professional role very seriously. I have found that this holds true even if the patient doesn't understand or accept the therapist's reasons. In some cases, a patient's offer of a handshake after a session that has been experienced as very productive will be a way of unconsciously testing the therapist to see if he or she will begin to take advantage now that the patient's defenses have been lowered. Of course, in other instances, a sudden offer of a handshake could be an indication that the patient felt relieved and understood during the visit.

Offering complimentary and supportive remarks.   In all psycho-therapy, and most particularly in the supportive modalities, it is considered appropriate for the therapist to provide positive feedback to the patient concerning his or her constructive attributes. The purpose of such interactions is to clarify confusion and investigate problem areas of self-esteem. Nathanson (1992) stressed the value of supportive remarks in the treatment of patients burdened by excessive shame. Many patients are fearful of acknowledging or enjoying appealing qualities that others notice in them because they perceive these qualities to be the source of intrafamily conflict or of exploitation. For this reason, many patients are totally refractory to compliments until they have gained a better understanding of the fearful associations that are attached to them. It is often tempting for a well-meaning therapist to tell a self-deprecating patient that he or she is physically attractive. The therapist may do this as a way of finding out more about the basis for the patient's beliefs, or to challenge the patient by implying that not everyone agrees with his or her negative evaluation. The patient might experience this as a sign of the therapist's personal defectiveness (i.e., "something must be wrong with anyone who thinks well of me."); as an indication that the therapist cannot tolerate the real problems because he or she is trying to seal over the bad memories connected with the patient's negative self-evaluation; or as a signal that the therapist is being seductive for exploitive purposes. For these reasons, therapists are well advised to employ complimentary feedback only after they have gained a better understanding of the reasons why the patient feels so negative about himself or herself. Praising something you do not understand is like signing a blank check and handing it to a stranger.

Searles (1959/1965) reasoned that it may be healthy for the therapist to acknowledge his or her feelings about the patient's attractiveness during the treatment process if this occurs in the context of the patient's accepting the impossibility of these feelings ever being enacted. Comparing the therapist-patient relationship to the oedipal triangle, Searles (1959/1965) noted that the incest taboo is maintained by

> deference to a recognizably greater limiting reality . . . the child emerges with his ego strengthened out of the knowledge that his love, however unrealizable, is reciprocated; and strengthened too out of the realization, which his relationship with the beloved parent has helped him achieve, that he lives in a world in which any individual's strivings are encompassed by a reality much larger than himself. (p. 302)

No matter how useful supportive compliments may be, therapists should be guided strictly by a realistic appraisal of their own limitations and of the patient's welfare. Patients tend to respond best to positive feedback that comes from a reality-based assessment. Such feedback should be clearly connected with something that has taken place in their own experience, or that has repeatedly been demonstrated within the treatment setting. For example, if a patient says, "I'm stupid; I never know what's going on," it might be very helpful if the therapist is able (from actual experience with the patient) to say: "I don't know about that, it seems to me that whenever I've made a mistake in our scheduling, you always have caught it and brought it to my attention."

Risky Forms of Physical and Emotional Involvement

Embracing, holding hands with, or kissing patients.   Freud's letter of December 13, 1930, to Ferenczi (Jones 1957), discouraging the latter's use of embracing and kissing as a form of "substitute mothering," embodies the classic argument regarding the riskiness of this type of physical intimacy. When utilized for nonclinical purposes, physical touching has the potential to arouse either party's expectation that the relationship will go beyond ordinary professional constraints. This hazard exists regardless of the clinician's speciality, but appears to be greater for those in the mental health field. In most circumstances, it would be harmless and probably supportive if, after performing a painful medical procedure, a family doctor placed a comforting hand on the patient's shoulder. The same behavior in a psychotherapy setting is likely to have a more complex meaning for patients because they don't usually come expecting physical care. A psychotherapist's work involves a special type of intrusion into the patient's *psychological* space. A treatment situation that combines a crossing of *both mental and physical boundaries* is probably too confusing for many psychologically disturbed individuals and should be segregated into distinct functions (Freud 1913/1958).

Certain attitudes and practices with regard to therapists' touching their patients might be gender specific. Perry (1976) reported survey results suggesting that female physicians (including psychiatrists) were *more likely* to believe nonerotic touching of patients to be therapeutically useful, yet *less likely* to advocate or engage in erotic behavior, than were male physicians. Holroyd and Brodsky (1977) found that 27% of therapists (Ph.D. psychologists) engaged in nonerotic touch such as hugging, kissing, or affectionate touching with patients of the opposite sex. Significantly more female therapists engaged in such contact with female patients than with male patients. Regardless of whether the physical contact was with a patient of the same or the opposite sex, it was endorsed more frequently by therapists with a humanistic orientation (25%) than by those favoring a psychodynamic (5%), behavioral (5%), cognitive (5%), or eclectic

(10%) approach. In a subsequent analysis of their survey data, Holroyd and Brodsky (1980) found that therapists who admitted to having intercourse with patients employed nonerotic touching with *opposite sex* patients more often than did other therapists. They construed these findings as an indication that gender-biased (heterosexual) touching is more likely to lead to sexual intercourse.

In the second factor derived from factor analysis of our Exploitation Index, we determined that touching patients (exclusive of handshake) loaded heavily with the following items: psychiatrist and patient addressing one another on a first-name basis, accepting gifts or bequests from patients, and joining with a patient in an activity to deceive a third party (Epstein et al. 1992). We interpreted the grouping of these items as indicating well-meaning but misconceived efforts to be friendly and ingratiating with patients. The fact that touching per se did not load heavily with a tendency to eroticize the treatment relationship tends to support Holroyd and Brodsky's (1980) findings that nonerotic touching does not always correlate with a higher risk for sexual exploitation. However, even if most physical touching never leads to sexual activity, it might be harmful in other ways (see Chapter 13).

At times, patients may surprise their therapists by suddenly embracing them either at the end of a session or during a crisis. This is best handled by calmly yet firmly setting limits:

> I can tell that you are having strong feelings about wanting to be close to me; we can best deal with this if you tell me what is going on in your mind; I am unlikely to be able to help you if these feelings are put into action.

This response imparts the message that there must be no exceptions in adherence to the therapeutic task. Patients who were sexually abused as children are particularly wary of a changing set of rules, because the offending parent would use exceptions as a way of rationalizing away the incest taboo.

Eating and drinking with patients. The tendency of some therapists to allow or even encourage patients to eat and drink during the therapy sessions appears harmless enough on its face. Nevertheless, this type of behavior tends to detract from the seriousness and purpose of the therapy. It is probably much more of a problem in longer-term psychodynamic therapy than in other paradigms. Problems arise because this behavior blurs the distinction between a therapist-patient relationship and the ordinary relationship between friends or relatives. Although sharing food or dring is usually well intentioned as a way of placing the patient at ease (it often succeeds in this regard), it runs the risk of sending the signal to the patient:

> This is just like any other relationship that you have been involved in.

Meeting with patients outside of therapy sessions.   Chance meetings between therapist and patient outside of the therapy sessions are quite common, particularly in small communities or when both parties are members of the same professional group. Planned meetings are probably less common. As previously cited by Borys and Pope (1989), between 7% and 11% of therapists admit to such encounters. We observed that only 1.7% of psychiatrists admitted that they actively *sought* contact with their patients outside of sessions (Epstein et al. 1992). The therapist has a responsibility to maintain professional boundaries and confidentiality by avoiding contact in such situations. Doing so requires considerable tact because of the likelihood that the patient will feel humiliated if there is a blocking off of his or her usual sense of what it means to be connected to another person. Avoiding contact outside of sessions should be reframed in a positive way with the patient:

> Ours is not an ordinary social relationship; rather, it is a special situation in which you are free to say whatever you wish to me. This requires a private and confidential setting. I want to be able to provide you with this kind of secure environment so that you will have the best chance of resolving your problems without intrusion and distraction. If my failure to acknowledge you in public stirs up feelings of shame or embarrassment for you, let's talk about it so that it needn't be so secret or fearful an emotion.

It is easy for a therapist who has difficulty dealing with his or her feelings of shame to assume that such things will be too humiliating for the patient to deal with. The temptation will be to treat encounters as ordinary social relationships for fear of offending the patient. However, this behavior may impart the following negative message to the patient:

> Shame is too awful a feeling to deal with or even to talk about. I'll just be nice to you so as to help us both avoid the topic.

Of course, other factors may play a role in chance encounters with patients. Some therapists will sense that a patient is too fragile to deal with the sense of hurt and rejection involved. This is particularly true when it is obvious that the patient knows the therapist has noticed his or her presence. In such situations it might be appropriate to briefly acknowledge the patient's presence if he or she has initiated a greeting and to discuss the issue at the next session.

The risk of meeting outside of the therapy session is that such encounters will lead both patient and therapist to become confused about the purpose of the relationship. Is it treatment or friendship? For example, Gabel et al. (1988) discussed the way therapists might handle a child or adolescent patient's request that they come to an important social function like a confirmation ceremony. These authors cautioned that therapists who accept such invitations might provoke unconscious competitiveness in the patient's family members and interfere with an opportunity to work with the child on his or her fears about the event.

If a clinician anticipates that an extratherapeutic meeting with a patient is likely, it would be wise to caution the patient that there should be no social acknowledgments outside of the treatment setting, since such contact might threaten the confidentiality and therapeutic nature of the relationship. Even in the absence of a prior discussion, in most cases it is reasonable for a therapist to avoid contact with a current or former patient in the event of an accidental meeting. The dynamics of chance encounters are such that unless the therapist goes out of his or her way to make contact, the patient is unlikely to initiate a greeting. Most patients will accept and appreciate this as a sign of the therapist's serious commitment to maintaining their privacy and confidentiality.

Having repeated and intense erotic feelings/thoughts about a patient.   Sexual obsessions and fantasies about patients are almost ubiquitous. Items loading on the first factor ("eroticism") found in factor analysis of the Exploitation Index survey were endorsed by approximately one-fourth to one-half of the respondents (Epstein et al. 1992). Criterion items on this "eroticism" factor included taking pleasure in romantic daydreams about a patient (33.2%); comparing the gratifying qualities observed in a patient with the less gratifying qualities of one's spouse (24.7%); experiencing a patient's seductiveness as a gratifying sign of one's own sex appeal (30.0%); and feeling a sense of excitement or longing in anticipation of a patient's visit (51.1%).

Prolonged and repeated fantasies about a patient may be a danger sign that a therapist is struggling with unresolved conflicts. This is most likely when the fantasies have an obsessive quality or feel more gratifying than troubling. The therapist's narcissistic conflicts can easily be exported onto a needy and vulnerable patient in the form of sexual imagery, teasing, and flirtation (see Chapter 3 regarding the "avoidance" and "attack other" defenses against shame). Even if the therapist's erotic fantasies never progress to actual physical involvement, they are likely to be communicated to the patient in a covert form. Vulnerable patients can be induced to act out their therapist's hidden wishes. Acting-out behavior sometimes occurs with a third person unconnected with the treatment who possesses certain characteristics that remind the patient of the therapist.

The therapist who experiences enduring erotic preoccupations about a patient should try to fathom the cause. It is risky to assume that the pleasure of being in the company of an exciting and attractive patient is merely a gratifying side benefit of doing psychotherapy. The therapist should endeavor to ask himself or herself questions such as the following:

1. Is the pleasure I am getting out of looking at this patient and/or enjoying the excitement of his or her presence leading me to forget what my job is?

2. What might my own feeling of falling in love or lust with this patient tell me as a communication about the way he or she loses a sense of control?
3. How is this patient's vulnerability or sense of shame similar to feelings that I too have experienced but would like to dispel?
4. Is the excitement of my "love/lust" for the patient a way that I (and the patient) seek to bury feelings of shame over rejection and disconnectedness?
5. Is the "god-like" feeling of having this patient adore me and idolize me the source of the erotic "rush" I feel with him or her?

The item concerning "god-like" feelings deserves particular attention. Some women have reported that their involvement with a former therapist was like having "sex with a god." The exploitive therapist may feel a corresponding "rush" of power and excitement. Fantasies of having absolute power over another human being form a key element in the fantasies and obsessions of sexually sadistic serial killers. Dietz and Warren (1992) described the motivations of one such offender who systematically tortured and raped women while he was slowly strangling them to death. He revealed the "dark secret" of how he achieved this strong exhilaration and pleasure:

> Let me tell you about sadism . . . the object is not to cause pain . . . pain is just a *way* of humiliating and being totally dominating over her . . . seeing the humiliation in her eyes . . . it is the supremacy of murder, the god-like ability to cause suffering . . . I enjoyed it so much I knew I had to do it again. (Dietz and Warren 1992, paraphrased quotation)

Contraindicated Forms of Physical and Emotional Involvement

Engaging in sexual behavior with current patients. This behavior has been repeatedly demonstrated to be harmful to patients (Luepker 1990). It constitutes a breach of the ethics of all major mental health professional organizations and is in violation of the statutes of at least seven states (see Table 1–1). R. I. Simon (1992b) emphasized that misuse of the transference is not the only basis for civil and professional sanctions against offenders. For example, a psychiatrist who applies a strictly biological approach could be sued on the grounds that he or she exercised undue influence on the patient or breached a fiduciary duty. The same principles would pertain to other therapists who do not employ interpretation of transference as a part of their treatment method. For a comprehensive review of the legal ramifications of sexual misconduct with patients, see Simon's chapter on undue familiarity (R. I. Simon 1992b).

Engaging in sexual behavior with former patients (posttermination). Although the issue of sexual involvement with *former* patients continues to stimulate considerable debate, the trend within mental health professional organizations has been to strongly discourage or proscribe such behavior.

For example, in standard 4.07 of the Ethical Principles of Psychologists and Code of Conduct of the American Psychological Association, psychologists are required to abide by a 2-year waiting period after ending treatment with a patient (American Psychological Association 1992). The code strongly discourages sexual behavior with former patients even after the 2-year interval, by emphasizing that it is often injurious to patients, and that it undermines public confidence in the profession. This code places a virtually impossible burden on any psychologist who would try to invoke the waiting period by requiring him or her to demonstrate that the sexual activity with the former patient is *not* exploitive.

Previously, the American Psychiatric Association handled this issue in its ethical guidelines as follows:

> Sexual involvement with one's former patients generally exploits emotions deriving from treatment and therefore almost always is unethical. (American Psychiatric Association 1989, p. 4)

In July 1993, the American Psychiatric Association removed all ambiguity in the matter by revising its position as follows:

Additionally, the inherent inequality in the doctor-patient relationship may lead to exploitation of the patient. Sexual activity
with a current or former patient is unethical. (American Psychiatric Association 1993, p. 4)

Appelbaum and Jorgenson (1991) have argued that there are
legal limitations to the right of the state to interfere with the rights of
individuals to freely associate with one another. These authors believe that a waiting period of at least 1 year should suffice in most
psychotherapy cases to protect a patient from exploitation by a former therapist. Appelbaum and Jorgenson's article stirred up some
very strong responses from other authors. In an example that tends to
prove the previously cited quotation (Gonsiorek and Brown 1990, p.
291) that "the half-life of the transference is longer than that of
plutonium," Spindler (1992) reported the case of a patient who was
devastated when she and her "former" therapist become sexually involved, even though that relationship was initiated more than 15
years after her apparently successful treatment with him had ended.
Brown et al. (1992) argued that exploitive therapists who are capable
of a certain degree of forbearance could easily employ a 1-year waiting period to "groom" a certain patient for a posttermination erotic
relationship. Gabbard and Pope (1989) reviewed the enormous hazards that are likely to arise for any therapist who believes this type of
practice to be acceptable. They cited the fact that posttermination
status has never successfully protected a therapist in a malpractice
case or disciplinary hearing, even though this point has frequently
been brought up as a defense.

In my opinion, legalistic arguments about permissible waiting periods ignore the fundamental purpose of the therapeutic frame. I do
not believe it possible for a therapist to conduct coherent psychotherapy unless he or she can *permanently* relinquish the prospect of *ever*
obtaining gratification from the patient for *anything* besides the contracted compensation. The treatment frame is a reflection of the
therapist's ego boundaries. If a therapist *seriously* entertains an actual
plan for sex with a patient after termination, it suggests that he or she
suffers from impaired ego boundaries. Such a plan would probably be
communicated to the patient *during the treatment itself,* and thus

would likely damage the treatment even if the scheme were never consummated.

In its *least* harmful manifestation, posttermination sexuality is closely akin to incest between a parent and a grown-up child. Most people realize logically and intuitively that it is just not a very healthy thing to do. Nevertheless, children and adults alike will find the most creative and legalistic rationalizations for justifying their attempts to gratify their incestuous wishes. Patients with such fiercely maintained impulses can be handled effectively only if the therapist remains tenaciously focused on the purpose of treatment. For example, in his book on the mutual story-telling technique for children, Gardner (1971) demonstrated how persistent he had to be with his patient. "Daniel" was a 12-year-old boy whose oedipal wishes for his mother were embodied in his fantasies of coming upon a cache of unearned wealth. As part of his therapeutic method, Gardner would match each of the patient's stories with a similar story of his own. Each rejoining story contained suggestions for how the characters in the narrative could deal more adaptively with their impulses and conflicts. The theme of "Daniel's" stories developed a more mature attitude as he made therapeutic progress. At one point, he told a story in which two boys wanted to buy a pair of bikes for a total of $150. The two boys "earned" $149.99 and then "found" the remaining 1 cent they needed to buy the bikes. Gardner remained the "cruel taskmaster" by insisting (in the matching story he told the patient in reply) that the two boys had to earn *all* of the money to purchase their bicycles. *Every last penny.*

The same message should hold for those of us who choose to become mental health professionals. Like Gardner's patient "Daniel," the therapist who allows himself or herself to become romantically involved with a former patient can be seen as having failed to relinquish that last remnant of the incestuously derived wish to "get something for nothing." The consulting room is advertised as a place for treatment. It should never be allowed to become a place to meet prospective sexual partners like a "free dessert" for the therapist to enjoy. Therapists who cannot relinquish this "last penny" are unlikely be able to help patients deal with their own incestuous conflicts.

Recommended Ways of Dealing
With Boundary Violations
Pertaining to Abstinence

Covert signs of violations of the rule of abstinence.   Therapists should be alert to changes in their own behavior that might foreshadow sexualization of the treatment (Epstein and R. I. Simon 1990; Gabbard 1991; R. I. Simon 1989; see also Table 12–1). The patient is likely to send covert signals of his or her own. Dreams may include scenes of doors being removed from hinges, of bugs coming in through the vents, or recrudescences of incest-related themes. The patient's associations might contain criticisms of other people in the patient's life who have exploited him or her sexually; anger toward people who cheat on their spouses; and grandiose images of being "special," such as a coronation. The patient may begin to act out by becoming sexually involved with an inappropriate partner.

Reparative responses.   If the therapist has engaged in preliminary seductive behavior that has not yet progressed to sexual contact, it may not be too late to salvage the therapeutic frame, provided that the therapist is able to stop the behavior and regain a proper professional stance. Even if the treatment has been irrevocably compromised, the therapist may still be able to acknowledge the inappropriateness of his or her actions, to help the patient explore his or her feelings about the breach, and to suggest appropriate referral sources for continuing treatment. Such responses could markedly reduce the patient's injuries and help him or her to regain trust in the idea that psychotherapy itself may still promote healing. In some cases where the erotic behavior is very limited and has not progressed to genital contact, it may be possible to repair the damage to the treatment with the original therapist. However, it is hard to imagine this to be feasible unless the therapist were taking vigorous remedial action through personal psychotherapy and supervision.

As I mentioned at the end of Chapter 5, before attempting a "confession," any therapist in this position should recognize that he or she might be in serious legal jeopardy and should consult an attorney in addition to seeking psychotherapy and supervision. I believe that it would be particularly destructive if the therapist tried to refer such a patient to his own psychotherapist (see Chapter 7; see also Dahlberg 1970). In my opinion, this would be a way of converting a potential disaster into a certain catastrophe. If the offending therapist's personal psychotherapist knowingly accepts such a plan, it is a sign of the latter's complicity in a collusive treatment frame. The offending therapist should question the solidity of his own treatment (past or present) and consider consulting somebody else. (Readers interested in learning more about the rehabilitation of sexually exploitive therapists should consult Abel et al. 1992; Celenza 1991; Gonsiorek 1990; and Schoener and Gonsiorek 1990.)

CHAPTER 13

Treating the Patient
Who Tries to
Exploit the Therapist

Clinical experience proves that it is really dangerous to be nice to
some people; they immediately repay such treatment with some
mean trick, and this is all the more remarkable because previously
they showed only indifference.

Edmund Bergler, *Psychopathology of Ingratitude* (1959)

No good deed goes unpunished.

Anonymous

The lion attacks the limping deer.

Zoology 101

Guiding Principles Regarding
Exploitive Patients

Many patients attempt to manipulate and use their therapists in nontherapeutic ways. Common examples of relatively minor breaches
include failure to pay the fee as agreed, attempts to extend the therapy session after the time is up, inordinate use of telephone calls as a
way of obtaining free therapy, frequent telephone calls at inappropri-

ate times, and efforts to "borrow" items from the therapist's waiting room. We found that 57.7% of the psychiatrists responding to our survey made exceptions because they felt sorry for a patient; 56.3% made exceptions because they were afraid a patient would become angry or self-destructive; and 67.9% acknowledged failing to deal with patient behaviors such as paying the fee late, missing appointments on short notice, refusing to pay for missed appointments as agreed, or seeking to extend the length of the session (Epstein et al. 1992). On factor analysis, we grouped these three items together into factor 3, which we interpreted as an indicator of "enabling" behavior. Scores on this factor correlated with male sex ($r = .19$, $P < .001$) and a humanistic or psychodynamic orientation as opposed to a cognitive, biological, or behavioral orientation ($r = .15$, $P < .001$).

More serious behavior includes cajoling the therapist to falsify insurance forms; threatening accusations of abuse as a way of pressuring the therapist to falsify medical records (Gutheil 1992); stealing prescription pads from the office; attempting to undermine the therapist and the therapy with offers of sexual favors, expensive gifts, or secret information; and sexually or physically assaulting the therapist.

Whatever the type of exploitation or intrusion, therapists often feel confused, used, and betrayed by the experience. Therapists naturally place a high social and ethical value on helping others. Professionals in a service industry aspire to give people what they ask for. It is therefore quite a shocking and humiliating experience to be "punished" when one was only trying to be "nice."

Many therapists are burdened with unresolved rescue fantasies. Freud (1910/1958) argued that the desire to salvage a person of "poor character," or to become indispensable to a powerful authority figure, was often linked to unconscious oedipal fantasies. Esman's (1987) review focused on the aggressive and narcissistically controlling aspects of rescue fantasies. Apfel and Simon (1986) emphasized that some therapists who become sexually involved with patients are reenacting an oedipally based rescue fantasy in which the parent of the opposite sex is delivered out of the clutches of the "evil" same-sex parent.

Novice therapists tend to deal with the anxiety that arises from uncertainty and inexperience by employing grandiose defenses elaborated as rescue fantasies (Jackson and Stricker 1989). More experi-

enced therapists may also have difficulty dealing with their own feelings of repressed shame, and cannot stomach "disappointing" a patient. This attitude results in a form of introjective identification in
which the therapist allows himself or herself to become a sacrificial
victim so as to protect against seeing his or her own feelings of de-
basement mirrored in the patient's anger (see Chapter 3 regarding
the "withdrawal" and "attack self" defenses against shame). Shengold
(1991) observed similar features in the spineless parents of a certain
type of narcissistic patient. These parents tend to shrink back in fear
when faced with their child's temper tantrums. Their children grow
up with an incapacity to love, and become preoccupied with rageful
and sadomasochistic fantasies.

Hill (1955) emphasized that therapists' overzealous desire to
"cure" often conceals an unconscious desire for superiority, domination, and control derived from a pathologically narcissistic wish to
achieve distinction through morbid self-sacrifice. He emphasized that
the etymological meaning of "cure" (Latin *cura*) derives from the
processes of *care* and *concern*, which should be distinguished from
hubristic efforts to remold a patient according to an inner schema of
perfection:

> The physician has considerable ability to interfere with and retard
> and perhaps prevent the recovery of the patient. He has at least
> some modest power to facilitate the patient's recovery. . . . In no
> sense is the physician a magical power. . . . He will discover time
> after time that his power operations aimed at the patient . . . winds
> up, as does pride, in a fall. (Hill 1955, p. 194)

In a similar vein, it is worth quoting the well-known 16th century
battlefield surgeon, Ambroise Paré:

> Je le pensay & Dieu le guarit. [I bandaged them, and God healed
> them.] (Doe 1937/1976, p. 122)

When patients violate the therapist's boundaries, they are usually
reenacting pathological expectations learned in earlier relationships.
Their exploitive behavior represents one of the deviant ways in

which they frame interpersonal connectedness. Although it is the therapist's role and responsibility to intervene in such situations, many clinicians are prone to "enable" the aberrant behavior instead. Unless the therapist is able to confront the issue in a timely way and respond effectively, the treatment is usually damaged by such behavior. In many cases, the therapist denies the seriousness of the problem until things get totally out of hand, and then inappropriately attempts to berate the patient for his or her ingratitude. At other times therapists will counter with exploitive behavior of their own. In the latter situation, the resulting breakdown of the treatment boundary leads to formation of a "mutual exploitation society."

Allowing the patient to exploit the therapist is dangerous for all parties concerned. Permitting such behavior sets a sadomasochistic tone to the relationship that may reinforce similar trends in the patient. This conduct also interferes with efforts to achieve a full understanding and resolution of the patient's psychopathology. On the other hand, a firm but caring way of confronting patients with their exploitive behavior gives the following defining message:

> It is important for people to take care of themselves. Since I am a person, and since I value myself, I cannot sanction any behavior on your part that would injure me. By taking this position, I am setting a role model that I hope will also help you to deal with persons in your life who try to exploit you.

Indicated Ways of Dealing With a Patient's Exploitiveness

Discussing all boundary violations with the patient as soon as possible. Patients test limits as a way of phrasing an "action question." For example, the therapist should confront the patient if he or she is late in paying the bill in a treatment where there is a payment deadline. If the therapist neglects to bring up the issue, the patient's associations might reflect his or her perception that the therapist is not serious about the rules, is lackadaisical, or is being seductive by making a special exception in the rules. Gabel et al. (1988) emphasized the importance of setting limits with child psychotherapy patients who steal toys from the therapist's playroom. These authors focused on ways that such behavior could be addressed as a therapeutic issue.

Conducting a post hoc check of the patient's associations and behavioral reactions to any boundary exceptions that are required as the result of an emergency.   Clinical exigencies require that therapists sometimes allow patients to impose upon them. For example, a suicidal patient may insist on being seen late at night or on a holiday. Some therapists are likely to experience such demands as intrusive and become angry at being "manipulated." To defend themselves against feeling weak, they will respond with an inappropriate posture of pretended invincibility: "Nobody is going to manipulate me."

Even if the patient is "only" being manipulative, the therapist, by assuming an overly defensive attitude, is unlikely to help the patient gain better control of his or her impulses. The patient can easily perceive such a reaction as a lack of care on the therapist's part. By displaying excessive counteraggressiveness, the therapist might provide the patient with an ill-gotten opportunity to turn the tables in a spitefully self-destructive "Gotcha!" maneuver (R. I. Simon 1992b).

Some clinicians have great difficulty dealing with the embarrassment and anger they feel in response to a patient's demandingness, despite clear indications that the behavior pattern is probably harmful to the patient, the therapist, and the treatment. These therapists may overcompensate with a passive, compliant stance that sets them up for repeated victimization. In the face of such a dilemma, it is important for the therapist to address the issue by carefully monitoring the pattern of manipulative behavior and developing a strategy for the nature and timing of interventions. For example, the therapist might have to "rescue" first and confront later. This approach deprives the patient of an opportunity for spiteful revenge and gives the therapist a credible standing when it comes to setting limits. Once the patient is clinically stable, the therapist is in a much stronger position to check out the patient's associations to the event and to address any exploitive component that might have been embedded in the patient's help-seeking behavior:

Mr. Tripp: (calling his therapist at 2:30 A.M. on Saturday): I can't stand it any longer, Doc, I don't think I can control these thoughts about going out and crashing my car.

Dr. Unger: Uh, er . . . how long have you been feeling this way?

Mr. Tripp: For the last few days, Doc . . . you've got to do something! I don't think this medicine's working.

Dr. Unger: Er . . . OK, meet me down at St. Willard's Hospital admissions right away.

[Two days later, housed on the psychiatric ward, the patient is feeling fine.]

Mr. Tripp: I got my car worked on last week. I change the oil myself every 3,000 miles, but I couldn't fix this rattle I heard under the hood. I go to this new mechanic. You just can't trust these clowns. So after he works on it, I drive fast down 43rd Street, er, you know, with all the potholes? I drive over this at 55 mph just to check out if I can't trust this joker to tighten all the rattles.

Dr. Unger: So maybe a few days ago you were checking me out, too, to see if you could trust me?

Mr. Tripp: Naw, you're OK, Doc.

Dr. Unger: Well I'm glad you think I'm OK, but do I have to get jerked around at 55 mph over a bumpy road just to prove it? . . . You know, I've noticed this pattern you have of pushing people and things to the limit, just to prove that they will let you down sooner or later. Maybe this is why you waited to call me late at night on a weekend to tell me how bad you were feeling, instead of calling me earlier.

Taking precautionary framing measures with patients who have a history of assaultive behavior or other types of predatory conduct.
A physical assault is the most serious violation of the therapist's boundaries. Such incidents are fairly common in inpatient settings, particularly in crowded units with a relatively low staff-to-patient ratio (Aquilina 1991). Whitman et al. (1976) studied 101 therapists from various disciplines. Of a total of 6,720 patients treated by the respondent clinicians during a calendar year, 9.2% appeared physi-

cally threatening to other persons, 1.9% appeared physically threatening to the therapist, and 0.63% actually assaulted the therapist. Bloom (1989) reviewed the literature on physical assault against therapists and found that between 32% and 61% of psychiatrists had been assaulted at least once in their career. When reported assaults were restricted to those occurring solely in outpatient practice, only 5% of practitioners reported having been assaulted by a patient, a figure that is no higher than the baseline rate for the respondents' non-work-related violence (Reid and Kang 1986). The nature of the patient's psychopathology and level of hostility seem to be the major factors in assaults against therapists.

The therapist's role in provoking or "inviting" an attack has not been well studied in a systematic and quantitative way. Some professionals appear more prone to being victimized than others (Aquilina 1991). Whitman et al. (1976) found that therapists queried about patient assaults were able to recall further memories of the incidents with follow-up interviews. Repeated discussion provided a useful catharsis for these individuals. Madden et al. (1976) surveyed 115 psychiatrists who reported being assaulted a total of 68 times during their careers. Of those respondents assaulted, 55% indicated that they thought they could have anticipated the attack and 53% thought in retrospect that they might have acted in some provocative fashion. Attribution of self-blame by victimized therapists must be interpreted cautiously, however, because it may represent a retrospective way of dealing with the helplessness elicited by one's failure to foretell a traumatic event (Epstein 1989; Terr 1983). "Postdiction" is converted into an after-the-fact "prediction," and is often quite unrealistic. Lanza and Carifio (1991) demonstrated the lack of objectivity underlying postassault assessment of attacks on mental health personnel. They studied the reactions of nurses to a questionnaire portraying an assault by a hypothetical psychiatric patient. They found that when the assault scenario involved a mild injury, respondents tended to blame the nurse-victim more than if the injuries were severe, even though all other circumstances of the hypothetical attack were identical. Causal attribution of blame to the victim was significantly related to the respondents' scores on a scale measuring their belief in a just world. Lanza and Carifio suggested that blaming the nurse for the assault was a way of holding on to a fantasy of fair play and justice. Thus, blaming a person for the misfortune that befalls him or her is a way of preserving one's own belief system.

Blaming is just as counterproductive in therapy situations as it is for nontherapists who are victims of criminal behavior. Efforts to help therapists prevent such attacks should focus on identifying patients at high risk and exercising preventive measures. Tanke and Yesavage (1985) found that thought disorder and "activation" measured by the Brief Psychiatric Rating Scale (BPRS) distinguished assaultive inpatients from those who were nonassaultive. Approximately one-half of the assaultive patients were judged to be "low-visibility," in the sense that they did not engage in a verbal attack just prior to physical aggression. The "low-visibility" patients scored higher on the withdrawal-retardation factor on the BPRS, compared with the "high-visibility" and control groups. A discriminant equation using BPRS scores was able to predict between 88% and 94% of "low-visibility" assaults.

Madden et al. (1976) emphasized how important it is for therapists to be attuned to any fear or anger that may arise in work with patients. Denial of these emotions interferes with the therapist's ability to directly address the issue with the patient before things get out of hand. The therapist's fear and anger may be the first signal (to the therapist) that the patient feels out of control and needs external behavioral limits, or that he or she requires appropriate medication for symptom relief.

Assaults on staff members may be the manifestation of a dysfunctional ward milieu beset by poor morale and splitting (Lion et al. 1976), as—for example—in a situation in which hospital staff fail to attend to the fears of certain personnel who are managing the day-to-day care of a highly disturbed patient. Other personnel may be unaware of the risk of assaultiveness because of poor intrastaff communication. In outpatient settings, certain violence-prone patients should not be seen alone. Some impulsive children become physically aggressive with their therapists and require firm limit setting as part of their treatment regimen (Gabel et al. 1988).

Other types of predatory behavior are seen in patients who have a history of writing bad checks or who have defaulted on debts with other persons. With these individuals, it is wise to frame the treatment on a "pay-as-you-go" basis. If the patient feels demeaned by this arrangement, his or her feelings can be profitably explored. In such cases, mobilizing the patient's healthy sense of shame and differentiating it from its pathological aspects may be the most therapeutic thing the clinician can do for the patient.

Some patients make sudden sexual overtures that take the therapist by surprise. For example, Shor and Sanville (1974) described a female patient who unexpectedly embraced her therapist at the end of the session. She began making thrusting pelvic movements. The therapist was able to place his hands gently on her contorted neck and to ask her: "What is this bad and painful feeling up here when you also are asking for closeness?" The patient released her grasp, collapsed in tears, and was able to talk about her use of sex as a way of getting "body closeness." Similarly, children who are victims of sexual abuse may unexpectedly grab the therapist's genitals during a therapy session or expose their own (Gabel et al. 1988). Whatever the age of the patient in such cases, it is important that the therapist set immediate behavioral limits. Although the therapist should certainly try to explore the meaning of the patient's actions, by itself this is often not enough. A sexually aggressive act on the patient's part should be treated with the same urgency and seriousness as a physical assault, even if the therapist does not feel physically threatened by the patient's behavior. In fact, it is even more dangerous if he or she finds the behavior flattering or amusing, while telling the patient to stop. If allowed to persist, such conduct can be quite dangerous for both therapist and patient because it might lead to false charges of sexual abuse. The patient might not be treatable in a one-to-one, office-based setting. If the therapist relies solely on verbal means to discourage sexually aggressive behavior, action-oriented patients might interpret this response as a signal that they just need to be more forceful.

Relatively Risky Ways of Dealing With Patients' Attempts to Exploit the Therapist

Allowing frequent exceptions. Gutheil (1989) cautioned that allowing repeated exceptions of treatment rules was a signal of escalating boundary violations. He warned that such behavior facilitated the fantasy of a "magic bubble" surrounding the therapist-patient dyad. Therapists who fail to address repeated exceptions for issues such as scheduling, duration of sessions, payment of fees, and inappropriate use of the therapist are inviting trouble. We (Epstein and Simon 1990) cautioned that unaddressed and repeated exceptions occurring in conjunction with romantic feelings for the patient could represent the prodromal signs of "falling in love." Therapists in this situation are at risk for becoming blinded to their patient's actual treatment needs. They are likely to start reframing the situation according to the rules of romantic courtship and self-gratification.

Avoiding confrontation because of fear of the patient's anger. Pa - tients with a significant narcissistic or borderline component to their psychopathology are usually burdened with serious problems in regulating feelings of shame-related rage. Therapists must employ tact, empathy, and proper pacing of the treatment if they are to help these individuals. However, for any coherent and rational treatment to succeed, certain boundaries must be respected by all parties concerned. If the therapist finds himself or herself avoiding confrontation when limits are trespassed because of fear that the patient will become enraged, a serious problem is brewing that will become harder to manage the longer it is avoided (see the vignette of Dr. Wu and Mrs. Vellum, at the end of this chapter).

Many therapists who have difficulty dealing directly with their patients' aggressive demands find themselves habitually trying to appease them. As previously mentioned in Chapter 12, the criterion items on factor 2 of our Exploitation Index (touching patients [excluding handshake], psychiatrist and patient addressing one another on a first-name basis, accepting gifts or bequests from patients, and joining with a patient in an activity to deceive a third party) (Epstein et al. 1992) suggest a well-intentioned effort to get the patient to be more kindly disposed to the therapist. The grouping of these items suggests that therapists scoring high on this factor—like those with high scores on factor 3 ("enabling")—will have a harder time setting limits on a patient's pathological demands, and that they might be unwittingly encouraging their patients to exploit them. As would be expected when comparing orthogonal factors, there was no significant correlation between high scores on factors 2 and 3. However, the possibility exists that the two factors are measuring different aspects of "rescuing" behavior.

Allowing frequent intrusions into one's personal "space."   Many patients are accustomed to sadomasochistic relationships in which one party inevitably abuses the other. These individuals will try to structure their involvement with a therapist in the same way. Their behavior may include frequent late-night phone calls, taking items from the therapist's office, intruding into the therapist's personal life by attempting to contact members of his or her family, throwing objects at the therapist, and engaging in aggressive attempts to have physical contact with the therapist. As discussed in the prior section on precautionary framing measures, this type of behavior requires a firm and unambivalent response. The therapist should be ready to tell the patient that treatment may not be possible under the established paradigm if the patient cannot conform his or her behavior to the requirements of the therapist's need for personal safety and privacy. Allowing such behavior to continue over an extended period of time encourages escalation. Consultation is advisable in such cases.

Contraindicated Ways of Dealing With Patients' Attempts to Exploit the Therapist

Colluding in illegal or unethical activity because of fear that confronting the patient will provoke his or her shame or anger.   Some therapists will inadvertently enter into collusive payment arrangements because they are afraid of antagonizing a patient. For an example of a therapist engaging in fraudulent behavior as a way to avoid dealing with a patient's anger, see the case of Dr. Percy and Ms. Oakes in Chapter 9.

We (Epstein et al. 1992) observed that 17.2% of the psychiatrists responding to our survey acknowledged joining in an activity with a patient in a way that may have deceived a third party such as an insurance company (see the previous section regarding avoidance of dealing with patients' anger). Colluding with a patient to deceive a third party is contraindicated not only because it is unethical and usually illegal but also because such a practice severely compromises the therapist's credibility and thereby destroys the effectiveness of the treatment. In much the same way that con artists entrap their victims by suggesting that they engage in a "minimally" dishonest act to harm a third party, some patients can capitalize on a therapist's complicity by blackmailing him or her into an escalating series of deepening boundary violations.

Colluding in any illegal or unethical activity because of a desire to hold on to an especially attractive or appealing patient.   Colluding with a patient to commit an unethical act spawns the TNT of psychotherapy. The whole mixture is volatile, unstable, and explosive. This is the stuff soap operas are made of.

Recommended Ways of Dealing With Boundary Violations in Which the Therapist Is Allowing Himself or Herself to Be Exploited

Covert signs of violations.   Early signs that a therapist is in danger of being exploited include a "magical feeling" on the therapist's part that he or she is going to "cure" the patient, a sense that the patient is so needy that the ordinary rules don't apply, fear/avoidance of the patient's anger, a prominent feeling of needing to "prove" his or her worth as a therapist to the patient, and a strong urge to make special exceptions for a patient.

Patient activities include making very flattering remarks such as "How lucky I am to have such a dedicated and caring doctor," an attitude of entitlement, strong criticism about other doctors who don't do enough for their patients, suspiciousness of the motives of authority figures, and anger about caregivers' not providing enough.

Reparative responses.   The following vignette provides an example of how one therapist became aware of making special exceptions for a patient out of a fear of the latter's anger:

Mrs. Vellum was almost always 10–15 minutes late for her twice-weekly sessions with Dr. Wu. Dr. Wu tried unsuccessfully to explore this with her. Inevitably, Mrs. Vellum would manage to bring up an "urgent matter" right at the end of the session, thereby exerting subtle pressure on her therapist to extend the time. Dr. Wu was reluctant to "cut her off" because the patient became so enraged at the people whom she felt had abandoned her. As Ms. Vellum had told her previously: "They lead me on . . . and then just when I think I might be able to trust them and feel safe, it's like they spit in my face." When Dr. Wu gently tried to end the sessions on these occasions, Mrs. Vellum's face would become flushed and her muscles would tense up. Her tone would became strident and angry. Dr. Wu fantasized that the patient was about to get out of the chair and hit her.

After seeking consultation, Dr. Wu realized that she was over-identifying with Mrs. Vellum's feelings of anger when she felt rejected. She remembered that she, too, tended to feel mortified and enraged when people let her down. At the next visit with Mrs. Vellum, she decided she would try to head the problem off by approaching it early in the session.

Mrs. Vellum: My mother is impossible, you can never count on her. She's never really there for me. Oh, she seems so sweet, but she's really just a wimp, and she never even stood up for me when my father would criticize me. She's *still* that way with him. My father is always demanding . . . she waits on him hand and foot, but if she asks *him* to do something simple for her like pick up the laundry, you'd think she had thrown water in his face the way he carries on about it.

Dr. Wu: Isn't that what you have been doing with me? By coming late to your sessions, you have arranged it so that you don't get enough from me and then you have to ask for more. And when the session is supposed to be over, I have been letting you take away from *my* time because you haven't gotten enough. In acting that way, perhaps I remind you of your mother who never puts her foot down. So I think I have been letting you down by not ending the sessions on time. I think it's important to insist that we stick to the limits of our schedule, even if it stirs up feelings that are very upsetting for you. If my announc-

ing the end of the session when you have still have something
more to talk about makes you feel demeaned and angry, I do
want to hear about it, but it's important that we wait until the
next session to work on it.

By obtaining consultation and conducting self-analysis, Dr. Wu
was able to repair the breach in the therapeutic boundary, to enhance
the patient's respect for her, to become a sturdier role model, and to
open the first real opportunity for work with Mrs. Vellum on her
shame-related rage.

Issues Concerning the Mental Health and Training of Psychotherapists

CHAPTER 14

Psychological Characteristics of Therapists Who Commit Serious Boundary Violations

Of incontinence one kind is impetuosity, another weakness. For some men after deliberating fail, owing to their emotion, to stand by the conclusions of their deliberation, others because they have not deliberated are led by their emotion.... It is keen and excitable people that suffer especially from the impetuous form of incontinence; for the former by reason of their quickness and the latter by reason of the violence of their passions do not await the argument, because they are apt to follow their imagination.

Aristotle, *Nicomachean Ethics* VII:7, 19–29[*]

The evils that befall man are of three kinds: The first kind of evil is that which is caused to man by the circumstance that he is subject to genesis and destruction, or that he possesses a body.... The second class of evils comprises such evils as people cause to each other, when, e.g., some of them use their strength against others...
. The third class of evils comprises those which every one causes to himself by his own action. This is the largest class, and is far more numerous than the [first and] second class[es].

Moses Maimonides (1135–1204 A.D.),
The Guide for the Perplexed[**]

[*] 1941 (ed. McKeon).

[**] 1956 (tr. Friedlander).

Qualitative Studies of the Psychological Characteristics of Erotic Practitioners

Most of the studies that attempt to explain the personal and psychological characteristics of therapists who commit serious boundary violations were drawn from clinical experience with offenders in forensic settings, supervision, psychotherapy, and the secondhand accounts of victims. Almost all of the studies have focused on practitioners who became sexually involved with patients.

Medlicott (1968) compared 18 professionals (4 were psychotherapists) who had committed "actual" erotic indiscretions with 12 individuals whom he judged to be victims of false allegations. He did not offer a rigorous set of criteria by which he distinguished the truth or falsity of the accusations. Of the "actual offenders," 11% suffered from a psychosis, 6% were neurotic, 44% had a character disorder, and 11% were alcoholic. Of the "falsely alleged" group, he found 82% to have no obvious abnormality, and 8% to suffer from character disorders.

Dahlberg (1970) presented nine cases of male therapists who became erotically involved with their patients. On average, the therapists were 20 years older than their patients (50 ± 7 versus 30 ± 6). One-third of the therapists were in the midst of separation or divorce. All but one of the patients were female. He found the therapists to be either depressed or sociopathic, and possessed of a tendency toward grandiosity. In general, they appeared as somewhat passive, shy, and introspective individuals who found themselves thrust into the tempting situation of having an attractive woman reveal her sexual desire. Dahlberg suggested that the therapists' erotic behavior represented the fulfillment of a long-standing fantasy nourished by many men, namely, an opportunity for sexual gratification without risk of facing the shame of rejection.

Marmor (1976) focused on the interaction between strictly situational features and therapists' characteristics in an attempt to explain sexual acting-out in psychotherapy. From a situational point of view, he found that the offending therapist is often a lonely, isolated individual suffering some form of marital disruption. He may be feeling deprived sexually in an unsatisfactory relationship. The patient is often a younger, attractive woman whom he perceives to be sexually available. From a psychological standpoint, Marmor (1976) observed four basic scenarios, the last three of which are most likely to be found in serial offenders:

1. The therapist acts out his projected needs to rescue a deprived and dependent patient by becoming involved with her sexually.
2. The therapist acts out what is essentially a nonerotic unconscious hostility based on a sadistic need to humiliate, exploit, and reject women.
3. The therapist acts like a "Don Juan." He repeatedly seduces women as a way of disavowing feelings of masculine inadequacy or conflicts over homosexuality. (These individuals frequently suffer from relative impotence or premature ejaculation. Their predatory compulsion for yet another conquest is founded on a need to "prove" their masculinity and sense of power. Women exhibiting a positive transference represent a quarry that these therapists seem unable to resist.)
4. The therapist has psychopathic features that he acts out with patients. (Individuals of this type are impulsive and suffer from a superego deficit.)

In Stone's (1975) report of his clinical experiences with erotic therapists, he described two psychiatrists in their late 20s whom he characterized as "disturbed" and "disturbing." These individuals were seen as "mavericks" by their colleagues. He diagnosed one as border-line and the other as sociopathic. Both had become enmeshed in pathologic rescue fantasies with seductive patients. Stone (1976) reasoned that "maverick" therapists are more likely to justify sexual behavior as an "innovative" form of treatment and to make exceptions to ethical rules because of their patient's "special" needs.

Apfel and Simon (1985) observed that in situations where treatment has led to sex, both therapist and patient appear to be involved in repeating an interlocking and complementary rescue fantasy. In one case, the therapist aspired to save a "damsel in distress" who was needy like his mother. In her early life, the patient had given ongoing support to her depressed father. This scenario was symbolically reenacted in the ensuing sexual relationship with her therapist, in which she was obliged to bolster his waning sexual potency.

Claman (1987) presented the case of a well-known instructor in psychiatry who enjoyed an excellent reputation among his colleagues until he was confronted by allegations of sexual involvement with several female patients. Residents in his teaching program were struck by his grandiosity during assessment interviews and by his penchant for detecting erotic transferences to himself by female patients. He became involved with one of his female patients who was also a former psychiatric resident. She idealized him and accepted his sexual advances because he told her he loved her and was tender to her at a time when she felt quite lonely. She reported the abuse after several of his other patients informed her that he had had sex with them and then rejected them. In Claman's (1987) other case, a female patient became involved with a prominent male psychiatrist. She had repeated intercourse with him because he declared his love for her and made her feel special and favored. She was shattered when she discovered that he had also been involved with other patients. She sought treatment from another therapist but felt ashamed that she continued to feel "under his [the first therapist's] control" and was unable to take legal action. Claman (1987) argued that, in ironic contrast to the idealized "true love" they profess to their patients, these therapists were seeking a mirroring selfobject to nourish a depleted sense of self. He explained the addictive and repetitive quality of their behavior by the fact that it is difficult to maintain such a fantasy with any one patient indefinitely. A needy individual seeking treatment for mental problems is unlikely to be able to reliably maintain her assigned role as a "mirror" for the therapist's "grandiose self."

Brodsky (1989) developed an impressionistic composite of erotic practitioners drawn from her experience with professional ethics committees, malpractice attorneys, licensing board investigations, and previous research on the subject. In her view, these practitioners are most often overconfident men who are disinclined to obtain consultations from other therapists. They may be admired as "gurus" by their patients and students because of their charismatic qualities. Frequently, these individuals believe that they are more talented than ordinary clinicians, and that their innovative techniques justify their disregard of the usual clinical standards. Their methods may involve extratherapeutic relationships and working with patients whom other practitioners are reluctant to take on.

Based on their clinical experience, Twemlow and Gabbard (1989) divided erotic psychotherapists into three categories. The smallest group consists of psychotic individuals whose behavior may be driven by delusional thinking. For example, one psychologist believed that God had commanded him to use his semen to bring eternal salvation to the teenage girls on his ward. A second, much larger group is antisocial. Therapists in this category ruthlessly exploit their victims and appear to show no remorse or empathy. The third group, estimated to represent approximately 50% of all sexually offending therapists, consists of neurotic individuals, those with assorted personality disorders, and those without obvious psychiatric disturbance. Twemlow and Gabbard (1989) characterized these therapists as "lovesick." Typically, they are middle-aged men who fall in love with younger female patients. Often burdened by problems with their significant others, these therapists present themselves as lonesome, needy, and emotionally defenseless to their patient-victims. Twemlow and Gabbard (1989) argued that the intrapsychic conflicts of these individuals could be best understood as arising primarily from dysfunction on a dyadic, selfobject level, rather then from the reenactment of an unconscious oedipal triangle. They emphasized that these therapists employ projective identification to export their shame-ridden feelings of vulnerability and disavowed femininity. These authors attributed the therapist's "nonpsychotic" and compartmentalized loss of reality testing to an oneiric trance-like state induced by the feelings of "boundaryless" union with the "selfobject" that has been projected onto the patient. Unfortunately, this idealized "love" conceals a perversion both of love and of the therapy that was promised to the patient. The therapist winds up injuring the patient by projecting his own feelings of humiliation onto her.

Averill et al. (1989) studied psychiatric hospital staff members who became sexually involved with their inpatients. They found that these male staff members could be divided into two groups. The first consisted of young men who were generally exploitive in all of their relationships. The second group comprised depressed middle-aged men who felt isolated, longed to be nurtured, and felt devalued or slighted by the institution in which they were working. Female of-fenders appeared to be trying to rescue the dependent and dysphoric male patients they became involved with, by healing them with love.

On the basis of their clinical experiences, Schoener and Gon-siorek (1990) found that most erotic practitioners could be classified in one of six clusters:

1. *Uninformed/naive*—These are individuals who have not achieved a proper education or understanding about the nature of profes-sional boundaries and responsibilities.
2. *Healthy or mildly neurotic*—These practitioners become involved with a single patient in a very limited way. They feel a sense of guilt about what they have done and will bring the involvement to an end on their own. At times they will turn themselves in. They do not repeat the erotic behavior with other patients.
3. *Severely neurotic and/or socially isolated*—Therapists in this group tend to become progressively involved with patients through ex-cessive self-disclosure and social involvement outside the therapy sessions. Any feelings of guilt that they might experience usually lead to self-defeating behavior rather than to self-restraint. These therapists often deny the destructive nature of their erotic activ-ity by focusing on the "love" that they feel for the patient.
4. *Impulsive character disorders*—These individuals frequently have a history of other types of boundary violations, such as defrauding insurance companies. Their sexuality has a compulsive quality. They also show an impaired ability to regulate sexual behavior in their personal lives, with students, and with staff members.
5. *Sociopathic or narcissistic character disorders*—In addition to having the compulsive/impulsive features of the previous group, these in-dividuals employ a more planned and cunning approach to the seduction of their patients. They are less prone to experience in-ternal conflict, and are more apt to use guile to prevent discovery.
6. *Psychotic or borderline personalities*—These individuals exhibit im-pairment in their reality testing and social judgment. They are

less likely to employ carefully rationalized excuses for their behavior.

Gabbard (1991) emphasized that erotic offenders who come for treatment usually do so because they are under legal and administrative pressure. Most often they either refuse to admit their sexual involvement or deny its damaging consequences. Gabbard (1991) found that only a small minority of these practitioners were suffering from overt psychopathy or severe narcissistic personality disorders. Nevertheless, he described a prominence of "narcissistic" themes in the "lovesick" therapists who comprised the majority of violators. Gabbard (1991) remarked that female offenders often enact a misguided attempt to rescue a "rowdy," impulsive young man from his "wayward tendencies." He argued that the latter scenario reflects a popular cultural theme in which an aberrant young man needs only "the love of a good woman" to settle him down. Most of the psychodynamic issues raised by Gabbard (1991) centered around therapists who suffered from problems of boundary confusion and self–other differentiation (see Chapter 12).

We (Epstein and Simon 1990) previously noted that some therapists who exploit their patients may be suffering from a psychiatric disorder—such as manic excitement, antisocial personality, or substance abuse—or from an organic brain disease that affects judgment—for example, dementia or frontal lobe syndrome. In certain erotic practitioners, repeated involvements with patients may indicate a paraphilic condition. In the latter group particularly, it is easy for the clinicians to deny the aberrant nature of their behavior because—on the surface, at least—their actions seem to fit into a normative pattern of mutual sexuality between consenting adults. However, recent work by Kafka and Prentky (1992a) suggests that men who engage in sexually compulsive behavior that bears a superficial resemblance to normal sexuality (nonparaphilic sexual addictions) share many comorbid features with paraphilic men who engage in more overtly deviant behavior.

Celenza (1991) presented a detailed case report outlining her analytic treatment of a male psychotherapist offender who had previously become sexually involved with a female patient. A key factor in this therapist's history was his childhood memory of witnessing his mother ridiculing his father. At the same time, his mother was seductive with him and treated him as her savior. He developed prominent grandiose defenses against a sense of narcissistic depletion and weakness. Much of this conflict was acted out when he violated his patient. He had perceived the patient as withholding, and felt that she needed to be rescued from her abusive husband.

More studies are needed regarding nonerotic boundary violations. As discussed in Chapter 9, violations involving money are probably more common than sexual transgressions. Geis et al. (1985b) collected a systematic sample of eight psychologists who were sanctioned for offenses against Medicaid. Allegations against the offenders included charges of filing false claims, fraudulent billing practices, and theft. All but one of the alleged offenders were highly resistant to accepting any personal responsibility for their legal difficulties. They blamed their problems on the bureaucratic inconsistencies and the inequity of the Medicaid program. Jesilow et al. (1991) presented several case vignettes of psychiatrists who were convicted of Medicaid fraud. They commented on the way that these clinicians employ self-deception, and the way their behavior arises from a "subculture of medical delinquency." These professionals rationalize their actions by invoking an ethos similar to the dyssocial group norms employed by juvenile delinquents—"Everybody does it, so it's all right."

Systematic Studies of the Psychological Characteristics of Boundary Violators

There is very little systematic data regarding the psychological characteristics of therapists who commit serious boundary violations. Existing studies have relied on self-report surveys that inquired about demographic factors and practice attitudes. Despite their limitations, however, certain inferences can be made from the available data.

Kardener et al. (1973) found that 17.9% of psychiatrists surveyed believed that erotic contact with a patient might be beneficial. Similarly, Holroyd and Brodsky (1977) found that 30% of male psychologists felt that erotic contact with a patient might be beneficial to the treatment, and 12.1% had actually engaged in such contact. The corresponding figures for female psychologists were 12% and 2.6%, respectively. Of those therapists acknowledging sexual intercourse with a patient, 80% had engaged in this behavior with more than one individual.

Gartrell et al. (1986) found that psychiatrists who acknowledged having sexual contact with patients were more likely than non-offenders to have undergone personal psychotherapy or psychoanalysis. One-third of the violators had become involved with more than one patient. Repeat offenders were less likely to seek consultation because of concerns about their sexual involvement. All repeat offenders were males. Overall, male respondents were 2.3 times more likely than females to be offenders. When asked about the reasons for their sexual involvement, 73% of the respondents cited "love" or "pleasure"; 19% indicated that their motivation was to help the patient's self-esteem and/or to give the patient a growth-promoting experience; 65% felt they were "in love" with the patient; and 92% felt the patient to be "in love" with them. One repeat offender initiated contact with 12 patients after the "termination" of treatment. He stated that his most recent sexual involvement started shortly after finishing treatment with the patient, and that he was "in love" with her. Comparing psychiatrists who initiated sexual contact during treatment with those who were involved with patients only after termination, the authors found that the posttermination violators were significantly more likely to believe they were "in love" with their patients, and significantly less likely to experience regret about their involvement.

Borys and Pope (1989) grouped therapists' responses according to 17 different items reflecting a variety of ethical attitudes about the proper way to deal with dual relationships and professional boundaries with patients. Questions focused on issues such as accepting gifts, accepting nonmonetary payment, disclosing details about one's personal stress, social involvement, and posttermination sexual contact. Using factor analysis, these authors identified three factors: 1) "incidental involvements," 2) "social/financial involvements," and 3) "dual professional roles." Several significant demographic contrasts were found with regard to factor-score loadings: for example, female therapists viewed involvement on the second and third factors as less ethical than did males.

Using multivariate analysis of psychiatrists' responses to our Exploitation Index (Epstein et al. 1992), we found several demographic characteristics that demonstrated a significant relationship to high boundary violation scores. These included male gender, private practice, and suburban practice location. Nevertheless, these variables explained only 16%–18% of the variance that placed an individual in a high-score category. For this reason, we concluded that demographic variables should not be overvalued as a predictor of boundary violations. Characteristics such as theoretical orientation, years of experience, and number of years of personal psychotherapy were not significantly related to high scores. We employed a nonlinear transformation of scores in order to correct for highly skewed responses, and found eight subgroupings of boundary violations on factor analysis. For example, respondents with high scores on factor 1 ("eroticism") were likely to be more preoccupied with the erotic aspects of their relationships with patients; those scoring high on factor 2 endorsed items reflecting well-meaning but misguided efforts to be ingratiating with patients; individuals scoring high on factor 3 ("enabling") seemed to have difficulty in preventing patients from taking advantage of them; and those with high scores on factor 4 ("greediness") appeared to have an inordinate concern for monetary advantage.

These studies suggest a need for further research to help define the differentiating psychological characteristics of therapists who become involved in serious boundary violations. Such information would be very useful in developing improved training for student therapists, and might assist in the rehabilitation and treatment of established practitioners.

General Psychodynamic Issues Found With Boundary Violators

Despite the limitations of our present knowledge, I believe it worthwhile to attempt to organize the evidence cited in the first two sections of this chapter in conjunction with other clinical considerations. In so doing, I hope to provide some useful generalizations about psychotherapists who are at the highest risk for committing boundary violations (see also Chapters 3 and 4).

Inadequate or improper training places a therapist at increased risk for committing boundary violations. Maintaining boundaries is a complex cognitive and emotional process. Individuals who have difficulty with ambiguity, uncertainty, and contradiction are more likely to rely on grandiose defenses and oversimplification as a way of reducing anxiety and cognitive dissonance. As mentioned previously, such individuals are more likely to violate their patients' boundaries. An adequate training process should help beginning therapists to identify these issues. It should also help those who cannot adapt to the ambiguity and stress of being a therapist to understand and accept their limitations. Not everyone who wants to do this kind of work is cut out for it.

Unless they have had some opportunity to work through the traumatic sequelae of their experiences, students who have been subjected to emotional, sexual, or physical abuse in their training or personal psychotherapy might be at greater risk to violate their own patients (see Chapter 15). These individuals are advised to have personal psychotherapy with a clinician who is carefully selected for his or her ability to maintain coherent boundaries.

A number of authors have emphasized the important role of narcissistic pathology in therapists who violate their patients (Epstein and Simon 1990; Schoener and Gonsiorek 1990; Twemlow and Gabbard 1989). We (Epstein and Simon 1990) reasoned that subclinical narcissistic conflicts were responsible for most of the psychopathology that underlies boundary violations. As a key feature of narcissistic pathology, maladaptive defenses against feelings of shame can play an important role in the way therapists manage therapeutic boundaries. These mechanisms may be present regardless of the presence or absence of actual DSM-III-R (American Psychiatric Association 1987) diagnoses such as narcissistic or antisocial personality disorders. In their quotation from Allen Wheelis's The Doctor of Desire (1987), a novel about a psychoanalyst who became obsessed with a talented female patient, Twemlow and Gabbard (1989) alluded to the manifestations of shame in their discussion of "lovesick" therapists who sexually exploit their patients in the course of falling in love with them:

> She is no other, she is I, In loving her I love myself, in rescuing her I redeem a part of myself—weak, frightened feminine—of which otherwise I must be ashamed. . . . I have found an idealized portrait of my hidden self. . . . My lovelorn enslavement is to a lurking image in a dark mirror. (Twemlow and Gabbard 1989, p. 82)

Wheelis's (1987) character bears some resemblance to the case described earlier by Celenza (1991). Disavowal of shame can lead to impaired ego boundary functioning, a segmented regression in reality testing, and the use of projective identification to export unbearable affects onto the nearest vulnerable target. Any individual incapable of mounting an adequate counterdefense—a child, a dependent spouse, an employee, a student, or a psychotherapy patient—is a likely prey.

The increased incidence of boundary violations among male therapists might be related in part to their greater tendency to use denial and projection as a way of regulating shame affects. This thesis is supported by Person's (1985) comments about the effects of gender on the manifestations of erotic transference. She reviewed the typical patterns of transference-countertransference phenomena in the four possible gender combinations (M-F, F-M, M-M, F-F) and concluded that the male therapist–female patient dyad is the one most likely to result in strong and conscious transference-countertransference feelings. Person postulated that this followed from the fact that men resorted to "power remedies" to defend against fears of narcissistic injury resulting either from lack of gratification or from being defeated by a competitor. She concluded that the gender distinctions in the differing manifestations of erotic transference among various gender combinations of patient and therapist could be linked to the fact that women tend to organize their identity around "defining relationships," whereas men accomplish this through achievement and autonomy. In employing maladaptive defenses against shame, male erotic practitioners are under intense pressure to enlist a social frame defined by sexual involvement as a conquest. Such a frame serves as a defensive way of feeling proud and masterful. Males are at particular risk for this mechanism because adolescent boys tend to receive peer group encouragement and approval when they boast about their sexual achievements with girls.

The phenomenon of the erotic psychotherapist as a grandiose, middle-aged male who is scornful of rules and prone to project his feelings of vulnerability onto others can be elucidated by Harder's (1984) research on self-esteem. Drawing from a nonclinical sample of college students, Harder (1984) found that subjects characterized as having "defensively high self-esteem" according to the research protocol scored lower on scales of perceived shame than did controls. He theorized that these individuals denied their conscious experiences of affects such as shame and embarrassment, and that they tended to be more boastful, aggressive, flamboyant, and histrionic. Compared with controls, the defensively high self-esteem students were more ambitious for achievement, attained a higher grade point average, were more self-centered, and had more frequent variation in their moods. They exhibited strong anxiety over the potential loss of cherished objects upon whom they depended for their self-esteem. These individuals also showed strong unconscious feminine identifications, against which they defended with hypermasculine attitudes. They needed to repress their feelings of shame as much as possible.

The authoritarian, parental role of therapist/healer has potent esteem-enhancing qualities that may be used in defensive ways to deny personal vulnerability (see Chapter 13). For example, Lansky (1992) emphasized the way in which men suffering from feelings of paternal inadequacy evidence strong denial of shame:

> These men will talk about almost anything rather than admit these failures at fathering. (p. 8)

Typically, these men struggled with the mortification they experienced around their own father's failure in the paternal role.

Because of defensive maneuvers similar to those observed by Lansky in "failed" fathers, "failed" therapists are impaired in their ability to regulate the minute vicissitudes of connections and interruptions in relationships. Pathological defenses against shame interfere with their becoming aware of the inappropriate nature of their bonding with their patients. Denial of shame also blocks this affect's valuable "signaling" function. Therapists who are not aware of their shame are more prone to engage in "shameless" behavior, to repeat their key traumatizing experiences, and to use projective identification to unload their disavowed affects onto their patients.

The stress resulting from any threatened cutoff of a valued emotional connection upon which a therapist depends for self-esteem regulation may lead him or her to regress to primary process thinking (see Chapters 3 and 4). Such a lapse is particularly likely if the patient's condition is refractory to treatment or if he or she has improved and is making efforts to separate. The therapist becomes threatened by this "differentiation" as a signal of impending loss, and seeks to reduce the distance by ignoring important boundaries. A vicious cycle is initiated in which the therapist may attempt to force his or her disavowed affects onto a dependent and defenseless patient. At the root of the problem is a defective configuration of the therapist's own ego boundaries (see Figure 3–7), such that he or she feels as if the patient is an integral part of himself or herself. The pathological deformations of the therapist's ego boundaries result in bilogical thinking very similar to that employed by incestuous parents (see Figure 4–3).

Certain narcissistic defenses against experiencing shame are frequently seen in therapists who are having boundary problems with their patients. As mentioned earlier in this chapter, the most prominent theme varies, depending on the phase of the clinician's career. Young practitioners will often employ grandiose defenses to deal with their uncertainty and inexperience. Middle-aged clinicians in their prime may become blinded to their patients' boundary needs because they have become overconfident and intoxicated by the success, recognition, and power they have achieved. As Henry Adams (1907) explained it:

> The effect of power and publicity on all men is the aggravation of self, a sort of tumor that ends by killing the victim's sympathies. (*The Education of Henry Adams*, Chapter 10)

Finally, toward the end of the therapist's career, his or her awareness of diminishing options, failing powers, and depression may lead to a parasitic desire to be rejuvenated by a liaison with a young and energetic patient.

Even when it appears in a subclinical form and in the absence of a comorbid mental disorder, narcissistic pathology will often result in a functional learning disorder or a segmental loss of reality testing. Traumatic memories of exploitation are often warded off by the encapsulation of a defensively overvalued ego state that erects a barrier through self-absorption, preoccupation with power, and the illusion of not needing others. New information that comes from another person can stimulate a threatening awareness of that other's separate existence. "Separate people" are unconsciously linked with "exploitive people who invalidate my existence." When a supervisor brings up new information that the therapist has never thought of before, or when a patient gives expression to his or her own unique and specific needs, these encounters may be perceived as terrible assaults upon the therapist's defenses because they provoke a painful sense of incompleteness, inadequacy, and humiliation. As a result, the "offending" information must be disavowed, ignored, or disproved, however vital it may be to the therapist's well-being. In this way, the therapist may become refractory to learning certain interpersonal information, even when he or she is earnestly trying to seek it out.

Another pattern previously mentioned in the literature review involves the tendency for offending therapists to become isolated from their colleagues. Such therapists may fail to pursue continuing education courses and tend to avoid obtaining corrective feedback from supervision. Even if they do obtain personal psychotherapy at some point in their career, the treatment frequently fails to deal with core issues connected with the origin of and defenses against overwhelming feelings of shame. An argument can be made that many talented therapists who later violate their patients have never had treatment in which these affects were systematically addressed. The whole topic of shame is one that has been relatively neglected in psychodynamic theory.

I have observed that therapists who become involved in serious boundary violations demonstrate a pattern of progressive denial of their failing powers. Their self-esteem is tenuously supported by narcissistic defenses. Such therapists will construct unbelievably elaborate mechanisms and justifications for their behavior as part of their efforts to deny their feelings of vulnerability and mortification. These mechanisms include rigidly constructed oversimplifications of complex clinical phenomena, idiosyncratic theories of behavior, and rationalizations such as "she was not my patient at the time" or "I was employing a different therapeutic model." Many erotic practitioners are in effect denying the incest taboo, as if one can obtain an exemption from rational civilized behavior by magically transporting oneself to an alternate universe in which such rules no longer apply.

CHAPTER 15

Education and Self-Assessment: How Can Therapists Learn to Improve Their Boundary Skills?

A teacher affects eternity: he can never tell where his influence stops.

Henry Adams, *The Education of Henry Adams* (1907)

Oh wise men, take care in your words, unless you be banished into exile to a place of evil waters, and your students who come after you will drink thereof and die.

Mishnayoth Nezikim, Avoth 1, Mishnah 11[*]

A person seeking to become a competent psychotherapist must absorb a complex body of professional knowledge and skills. The student's ego boundaries are expanded and strengthened during this process. He or she develops a "professional self" that embodies a new identity, that of a responsible caregiver. Reading and lectures

---

[*] Blackman (tr.) 1965.

alone are insufficient. If trainees are to become full-fledged clinicians, they must undergo a fundamental change in their way of relating to the vulnerable individuals who will come under their care. For this reason, there is no substitute for carefully monitored clinical experience. It is a supervisor's role to guide students on this path. A supervisor's message is transmitted through words, attitudes, and deeds. Such teachers are the idealized role models from whom students develop a coherent sense of the responsibilities and techniques that are necessary in patient care. The boundaries of the "professional self" that are acquired during training provide the foundation for the integrated treatment framework that the new therapist will employ in his or her work. If the supervisor's attitudes and behaviors are deviant or exploitive, it is highly likely that those attitudes will be assimilated as serious defects in the students' developing therapeutic ego boundaries.

There is a growing realization among clinical investigators working in the field of therapeutic boundary violations that a need exists for improved training methods for psychotherapists. Many professional organizations, teaching institutions, and individual clinicians have developed innovative approaches in recent years as part of an effort to educate therapists in boundary maintenance. This effort is undoubtedly an outgrowth of the perception that traditional methods of teaching and supervision have allowed too many colleagues to "fall through the cracks."

In this chapter I provide a review of some of the recent literature on the training of psychotherapists. My summary is organized around three major subtopics: 1) the problem of adverse role modeling that occurs when educators become sexually involved with their psychotherapy students, 2) recent proposals for improved training in dealing with therapeutic boundaries, and 3) the use of self-assessment methods to assist established therapists in their continuing education.

Importance of Detecting Adverse Role Modeling and Abusive Teaching Methods

In designing programs for teaching a subject as varied and complex as psychotherapy, it is evident that a great deal of the material is experiential and cannot be imparted by didactic methods alone. After deciding what it is we seek to teach to our students, it is important to ask ourselves: "What is the professional model that I wish to impart to them?" Words and behavior need to be reasonably congruent. A teacher who assumes a tactless, scornful, or demeaning attitude is sending an embedded message that may be consciously or unconsciously incorporated into the student's "professional self." A shaming message might proceed as follows:

> Look here, what psychotherapy is about is power. I am more powerful than you, so I can take away your personal sense of feeling worthwhile any time I choose. I have the knowledge you need for success, so you had better listen to me and obey or I will destroy you psychologically.

Teachers imparting this message are demonstrating how to use arrogance as a way to dispel shame and vulnerability. Students exposed to this type of defense are likely to employ a similar protective mechanism in dealing with their future patients.

When a supervisor engages in a sexual relationship with a student, a similar subliminal message is being sent:

> I am a powerful and important person and you need me. The prerogatives of power are such that I can get gratification in a way that ordinary people can never hope for. Not only do I want you to worship me, I also want you to gratify me sexually. Being a powerful person as a psychotherapist means getting admiration and sexual pleasure from people who depend on you.

Students incorporate such messages in varying ways. Those who cannot marshal an effective defense against such abuse are at great risk of assimilating these framing statements into the structure of their therapeutic ego boundaries.

Sexual involvement between teachers and students has been declared to be unethical behavior by most mental health professional organizations. For example, Section 4, Annotation 14, of *The Principles of Medical Ethics With Annotations Especially Applicable to Psychiatry* (American Psychiatric Association 1993) states:

Sexual involvement between a faculty member or supervisor and a trainee or student, in those situations in which an abuse of power can occur, often takes advantage of inequalities in the working relationship and may be unethical because: (a) any treatment of a patient being supervised may be deleteriously affected; (b) it may damage the trust relationship between teacher and student; and (c) teachers are important professional role models for their trainees and affect their trainees' future professional behavior. (p. 7)

In large part, professional societies have revised their ethical guidelines in response to a growing body of literature that quantifies the extent of abusive teaching practices in psychiatry and psychology training programs. A review of some of these data documents the rationales presented by those who believe that a need exists for change in our approach to students.

Sexual Involvement Between Students and Educators

The first area of study involves the question of educators becoming sexually involved with students. Pope and Bouhoutsos (1986) re-marked that whole "dynasties" of therapists and students exist who have transmitted a dysfunctional mode of relating both to their pa-tients and to successive generations of students. In a national survey of psychologists (Pope et al. 1979), 3% of the men and 17% of the women reported that they had been involved sexually with an educa-tor during their training. Educators included psychology teachers, clinical supervisors, and administrators. Of the women who reported such contact with educators, 23% also acknowledged that they had subsequently become sexually involved with one of their own pa-tients or students. Only 6% of female psychologists who had not been sexually involved with an educator reported engaging in erotic prac-tices with patients or students. This difference was statistically signif-icant. Sample size prevented significance testing of this issue for men.

Glaser and Thorpe (1986) queried female psychologists about sexual involvement with educators during graduate training. In their survey, 17% admitted to having been involved in such behavior. In retrospect, 36% of the respondents reported having thought that the sexual behavior presented both professional and ethical difficulties at the time it occurred. When asked how they felt about that behavior at present, 56% now felt that it presented ethical and professional problems. When asked about their "at-the-time" judgment regarding how much pressure they felt to cooperate with sexual advances from their educators, 71% reported their teachers' behavior as coercive. Of those respondents who refused sexual advances that were made to them by teachers, 45% indicated that they felt that they were punished to some degree as a result of this rebuff. In 7% of those who felt they had been punished, the retaliation was described as "strong."

In a survey of fourth-year psychiatric residents by Gartrell et al. (1988), 4.9% of the 546 respondents reported that they had been sexually involved with their educators. The latter included supervisors, instructors, advisers, and administrators. None of the 0.9% of residents who reported that they had become sexually involved with patients had been involved with an educator.

Carr et al. (1991) surveyed all psychiatric residents in Canadian teaching programs. In their study, 4.1% of female residents and 1.2% of males reported sexual involvements with educators. In the case of female residents, 9.7% reported sexual harassment by an educator during training.

All of the studies cited thus far inquired about psychotherapists' memories of sexual involvement with faculty members teaching in their graduate training programs. Tabachnick et al. (1991) approached the problem from another perspective—that of the educators themselves. Their survey respondents consisted of faculty members of teaching institutions, and represented all of the major branches of psychology. Approximately 11% indicated that they had become involved with a student. Similarly, 28% indicated that they felt that sexual involvement with a student presented no ethical problems.

Sexual Involvement Between Students and Personal Psychotherapists

A second major area of study has focused on the fact that a student's personal psychotherapy plays a crucial role in his or her ability to maintain a coherent sense of professionalism and to develop well-functioning therapeutic ego boundaries. Gartrell et al. (1986) studied this issue in a national survey of psychiatrists. They found that 1.6% of respondents reported having had sexual contact with their own psychotherapists. Two of those respondents were men who had subsequently also engaged in erotic practices with their own patients. Female psychiatrists were almost five times (4.4% versus 0.9%) more likely to have been involved with their personal therapists than were males.

Table 15–1 summarizes the findings of the studies on sexual involvement between students and educators or therapists.

Table 15–1. Summary of studies regarding sexual involvement between student psychotherapists in training and their educators

Authors/Population studied	Men (%)	Women (%)	Both (%)
Pope et al. 1979			
Psychologists in training			
Sexually involved with an educator	3.0	16.5	
Glaser and Thorpe 1986			
Psychologists in training			
Sexually involved with an educator		17.0	
"Punished for refusing involvement"		45.0	
Gartrell et al. 1988			
Fourth-year psychiatry residents			
Sexually involved with an educator	3.9	6.3	
Carr et al. 1991			
Psychiatry residents			
Sexually involved with an educator	1.2	4.1	
Sexually harassed by an educator	0.0	9.7	
Tabachnick et al. 1991			
Psychology educators			
Sexually involved with a student			11.0
Thought the behavior ethical			28.0
Gartrell et al. 1986			
Psychiatrists			
Sexually involved with psychotherapist	0.9	4.4	1.6

Abusive Educational Methods

A third relevant theme that has been documented in the literature focuses on educational methods that employ ridicule, shaming, and a general misuse of power. This problem remains latent in many health care training programs. Silver and Glicken (1990) reported that 80.6% of the students at one major medical school indicated that they had been subjected to abusive treatment within that institution by the time they became seniors. Reported abuse included repeated verbal shaming by teachers, sexual harassment, physical assault, and institutional neglect. For example, one female respondent from their study stated:

> ... this was not so much one major event as repeated ones: daily insults, rude remarks, etc., which went on for the entire 6 weeks and had a significant detrimental effect on my self-confidence for some time afterward.... I was told I was worthless... when I did answer correctly, I was never praised but was told that the stupidest of medical students should, after all, know this information.... (Silver and Glicken 1990, p. 530)

Sheehan et al. (1990) obtained a cross-sectional survey of the third-year class of an entire medical school that inquired about abusive behavior on the part of educators. Approximately 85% of these students reported that they had been subjected to humiliation and belittlement; 10% reported threats of physical harm by residents or clinical faculty; 44% reported being placed at unnecessary medical risk; 81% of the women reported being subjected to sexist slurs; and 55% of the women reported being the object of sexual advances, primarily by clinical faculty, residents, and interns.

Richman et al. (1992) conducted a prospective survey of abuse of medical students over the entire 4-year period of one class. Fifty-four percent of the students reported being "yelled at," 24% reported being "sworn at," and 4.8% reported being physically hit by faculty or house officers. Being sworn at or yelled at led to a significantly increased level of problem drinking and hostility over baseline measures recorded at the beginning of training. Analysis of covariance controlled for initial levels of psychopathology. Being hit was associated with increased levels of depression, hostility, and anxiety at the time of follow-up. When compared with measures for nonphysically abused students, these results were highly significant statistically.

Studying the educators themselves, Tabachnick et al. (1991) reported that 15.5% of psychologists whose primary work was in an institution of higher learning acknowledged having insulted or ridiculed a student in his or her presence. Similarly, 34.8% believed that it was sometimes ethical to engage in such behavior.

Table 15–2 summarizes the studies regarding the abuse and shaming of health care professionals during training.

I would suggest that predominantly male-dominated academic faculties have traditionally used ridicule and sarcasm as an embedded message in "motivating" trainees. This hypercompetitive, shame-driven institutional frame probably exacerbates the problems that so

Table 15–2.   Summary of studies regarding abusive and shaming behavior of health care students by educators

Authors/Population studied	Women only (%)	Men and women combined (%)
Silver and Glicken 1990		
Medical students		
Subjected to verbal shaming and harassment		80.6
Sheehan et al. 1990		
Third-year medical students		
Subjected to abusive behavior		85.0
Subjected to sexual advances	55.0	
Richman et al. 1992		
Medical students		
"Yelled at" by educators		54.0
"Hit" by educators		4.8
Tabachnick et al. 1991		
Psychology educators		
Insulted or ridiculed a student (in his or her presence)		15.5
Believed it ethical to do so		34.8

many vulnerable therapists in training encounter in their efforts to build a coherent sense of professional self-esteem. The role of shame in this kind of behavior is suggested by a reluctance to talk about the socially aberrant activity involved. One of the most common defenses against "feeling ashamed" is to attempt to hide or conceal oneself, embodied in the wish to "crawl under a rock" or to keep the whole event a secret (see Chapter 3 for a discussion of the "withdrawal" defense). Pope et al. (1979) may have documented this unwillingness to reveal a shaming event in their examination of the differences between early and late responders to their survey. It is reasonable to hypothesize that early responders were less defended against revealing a painful experience. The authors found that those psychologists who were late responders to the survey were more than three times more likely than the early responders to report having had sexual contacts with their teachers when they were students, and almost four times more likely to admit to having had sex with their own students or patients.

A special form of adverse role modeling occurs when psychotherapy training institutions require trainees to enter personal "training" psychotherapy with faculty members who also have an administrative responsibility to report on the students' "progress." Langs (1984–1985b) argued quite forcefully that, by depriving students of the protection of full confidentiality, this practice undermines their psychotherapy and teaches a corrupt lesson about maintaining a coherent treatment framework.

There is ample evidence from all of these studies to indicate that our training methods for psychotherapists need improvement. The teacher or psychotherapist of a student in training to become a mental health professional has the opportunity and privilege of transmitting a valuable healing method. He or she also has the power to pass on a destructive seed that can harm the student's professional identity—and thereby adversely affect successive generations of patients and students. As a consequence of this responsibility, it is essential that teachers and therapists who treat students have a thorough understanding of their own problems in dealing with boundaries, and of the defensive means they use in dealing with feelings of shame.

Review of the Literature on Educational Methods for Teaching Therapists About Keeping Boundaries

A number of studies have reported that professional training programs devote inadequate attention to the problem of boundary maintenance. Pope et al. (1986) surveyed 575 psychologists regarding the training they received to assist them in dealing with sexual feelings toward patients. One-half of the respondents indicated that they had received no training on this subject. Only 9% of respondents believed that the training they had received was adequate. Similarly, Glaser and Thorpe (1986) found that only 12% of their psychologist respondents indicated having received any training on the subject of sexual involvement between students and educators, or between therapists and patients. Pope and Bouhoutsos (1986) argued that more attention should be given to examining the personal and professional values of students admitted to psychotherapy training programs, and that more educational resources should be dedicated toward helping students achieve a better definition of therapeutic ethics and boundary maintenance. Gartrell et al. (1988) reported that only 12% of the fourth-year psychiatric residents that they surveyed in a national study indicated that therapist-patient sexual issues had been thoroughly discussed during their training. Residents who reported having addressed issues of sexual attraction to patients with their supervisors were also more likely to have had education regarding therapist-patient sexual contact in their programs. Residents who had been given some education about educator-resident sexual contact were more likely to have discussed their sexual feelings about patients with their supervisors than were residents who had not received such training.

As a result of these findings and in response to the growing public and professional awareness of psychotherapist-patient boundary violations, many groups have suggested specific improvements in educational methods. Although the recommendations and the techniques they employ may vary according to the treatment setting, a number of common themes recur.

Averill et al. (1989) developed an educational approach to help staff members on psychiatric inpatient units cope better with boundary issues. These authors believe that psychopathic individuals are unlikely to benefit from instruction in this area, and attempt to screen out such persons by preemployment interviews and checks for prior criminal records. New staff receive an orientation on boundary issues and patient-staff sexual relationships. The issue of touching patients is handled by focusing on the limits that are necessary when physical contact is required. Videotapes and pertinent literature on boundaries and staff-patient relations are provided to new employees. Periodic educational meetings and in-service presentations foster a sense of openness among the staff that makes it easier for them to talk about boundary issues and sexual feelings. The clinician team leader is encouraged to facilitate this process by discussing his or her own feelings about patients in a candid way. The leader's frankness tends to assuage staff members' fears of disapproval. Staff are taught about the danger of keeping collusive secrets in a ward atmosphere, and about the way such secrets might signal incipient boundary violations. Particularly vulnerable patients are identified by tactful inquiry about prior abuse and exploitation in childhood as well as sexual involvement with previous care providers.

Gafner and Trudeau (1990) developed a "Boundaries" workshop designed to assist mental health practitioners in the Veterans Administration system. This program was organized in response to a tragedy that occurred after a psychiatric nurse married a disabled veteran who had been diagnosed with chronic alcoholism and borderline personality disorder. This nurse had met her husband when he was a patient under her care on an inpatient unit. A year later, he shot and killed her and her two grandchildren. Gafner and Trudeau (1990) also developed a 10-item questionnaire for this workshop to assess both precourse attitudes and postcourse change in attitudes. In the workshop, small groups (three to five persons) discuss issues such as doing business with patients, giving or receiving monetary gifts from patients or their family members, and sharing a home with a patient.

Lazarus and Sharfstein (1992) reported that the American Psychiatric Association spends approximately $1,000,000 per year in connection with ethical complaints against its members. They found that 113 members had been expelled or suspended in the past 10 years, primarily for sexual misconduct with patients. To deal with this problem, the American Psychiatric Association has developed courses and videotapes on the topic of ethics and the problem of sexual misconduct. The American Psychiatric Association provides brochures and videotapes to help psychiatrists learn more about these problems. They also have prepared a "Fact Sheet" (American Psychiatric Association 1992) that is available to the public. This pamphlet is designed to educate laypersons about the dangers of patient-therapist sexual contact. It also provides a checklist of danger signs that might alert patients to the fact that their therapist is being exploitive. For example, patients are cautioned to be wary if their therapist engages in any of the following behaviors:

1. Discloses excessive and detailed information about his or her personal or sexual experiences.
2. Offers to waive or reduce fees when payment is not a hardship.
3. Offers to socialize outside the office or office hours.
4. Uses touch in "comforting ways."
5. Regularly begins to extend therapy sessions by 10–15 minutes or more.
6. Suggests a nontherapeutic relationship such as a business deal or soliciting stock market advice.

Gorton and Samuel (1992) presented their work in developing a new training approach for psychiatric residents at Thomas Jefferson University Hospital in Philadelphia, Pennsylvania. As part of their effort, they surveyed the directors of psychiatry and psychology training programs throughout the United States to find out what was being taught on the subject of therapist-patient sexual exploitation ($N = 196$; 69.4% return rate). Between 55% and 78% of responding programs reported including the following issues in their training curricula: current ethical guidelines (78%), managing eroticized transferences (75%), avoiding boundary violations (58%), and legal (56%) or professional (55%) sanctions against violators. More than half (55%) of the programs also stressed the value of personal psychotherapy or psychoanalysis for the student therapist. In most programs, these topics were taught in group discussion. Lectures, assigned reading, and individual supervision on the topic were used in less than half of the programs. Other modalities more rarely employed included case presentations, group viewing of videotapes, grand rounds, journal clubs, administrative meetings, role playing by residents and faculty, and victim-advocate presentations. Of all reported training programs on prevention of boundary violations in the survey, 55% had been in place for 4 years or less, while only 25% had been in place for more than 10 years. Gorton and Samuel (1992) proposed a 12-session model didactic course for therapists in training that would include lectures on ethical and legal issues, role playing in a mock trial, work on distinguishing between intrapsychic experience and the realm of action, use of self-assessment methods, group viewing of videotapes on boundary violations, discussion of case material, presentations given by victims, presentations given by a therapist-perpetrator, and discussion of the resident's own case material. These authors also suggested an integrated approach to the subject that would consist of material presented by both male and female faculty members over a 4-year period in a variety of formats within the total residency curriculum. This training would then be anchored by a core intensive course offered in the fourth postgraduate year.

The Massachusetts House of Representatives Committee on Sexual Misconduct by Physicians, Therapists, and Other Health Professionals (1992) sponsored a major conference on the subject of training therapists to prevent sexual misconduct and the abuse of power. As part of the curriculum subcommittee report for these meetings, Benson et al. (1990/1992) presented a working paper summarizing many of the pertinent issues that educators must face. They emphasized the importance of focusing on both the social and the professional contexts in which sexual misconduct occurs. In their paper, Benson et al. pointed out that insufficient study has been devoted to the way that offenders' behavior relates to the group dynamics of professional organizations, and they raised the possibility that offenders might be playing a scapegoat role for issues that are disavowed by their colleagues.

Benson et al. (1990/1992) also conducted an informal survey of psychotherapy teaching programs representing the major mental health disciplines in the Boston metropolitan area. In the survey, they inquired about the mechanisms employed by these programs to help students deal with sexuality and ethical decision making. Their results showed that a variety of approaches to this problem exist. Some programs focused on the way that teachers' sexual harassment of students could be connected with those students' subsequent sexual misconduct with patients. Others emphasized the modeling of professional ethics by striving for a thoroughly professional teaching environment. Still other programs held faculty meetings and workshops on the abuse of the supervisory relationship and the way such abuse relates to the use of self and power in the student-teacher dyad. Finally, several programs used role playing and case material to illustrate the management of ethical conflicts.

Benson et al. (1990/1992) emphasized the way in which the hypotheses one holds about the origin of professional sexual misconduct influence one's approaches to training and prevention. One teacher participating in their group discussion reasoned that sexual abuse of patients follows as a result of professional incompetence, and recommended proper training as a solution. Others felt that abuse of patients results from therapists' feelings of entitlement and unwarranted belief in their own privilege. These participants argued that students should be observed for subtle signs such as feelings of specialness or of believing that they are above the rules. Situational factors such as aging, loss of a loved one, and occupational stress were also suggested as important issues to be monitored. Other aspects considered to be conducive to sexual misconduct were the regressive pull of the psychotherapy process and the relative isolation of psychoanalytic practice.

New teaching methods suggested by participants in the Benson et al. (1990/1992) panel to address these problems included reviewing in detail the code of ethics of one's professional organization, using case histories of sexual misconduct to teach students, and employing small-group training to help establish a group frame for the ethical norms of professional behavior. Opinions varied considerably among the discussants regarding the ideal timing for introducing these issues into the training curriculum. Many participants felt that much depended on the emotional commitment of the faculty to the values being taught, and that teachers who are uninterested in this issue are also likely to be resistant to any change in the curriculum. Some participants believed that it was important for teachers to be able to expose their own vulnerability by revealing problematic experiences with patients. Such frank disclosure would demonstrate to students that it is safe for them, too, to admit to uncertainty and confusion regarding their patients.

At Georgetown University School of Medicine, I have participated as a faculty member in the training instituted by Dr. Robert Simon as part of his program on Psychiatry and Law. Psychiatric residents participate in a series of seminars focusing on the clinical and legal aspects of therapeutic boundaries. This training gives them an opportunity to learn about the way that the law views the psychotherapist-patient relationship in such key areas as informed consent, confidentiality, billing, sexual contact, and undue familiarity. Participants are able to discuss these issues as they pertain both to their professional relationships and to the current problems they may be experiencing with their own patients.

It is evident from the foregoing review that we have much to learn about improving our educational methods regarding boundary violations. Given our present state of knowledge, a multilevel approach appears to be the most sensible. This approach could include methods such as clarification of ethical guidelines for both faculty and students; careful screening and monitoring of faculty and students; traditional academic presentations on the clinical and legal ramifications of boundary issues; consciousness raising for all participants through discussion groups; and case seminars employing presentations of the experiences of faculty, students, victims of abuse, and rehabilitated perpetrators. These methods could serve as valuable supplements to a student's personal psychotherapy and the standard training curriculum.

Self-Assessment Methods

In this final section, I think it would be helpful to outline some of the ways that therapists can educate themselves about the problems arising from violations of professional boundaries. It appears to be part of human nature to overlook deficiencies in our training or technique. Requirements for continuing education programs among health care workers stem from an understanding of this tendency as well as from the fact that our healing skills can be maintained only by a lifetime commitment to learning. Perhaps the most important negative consequence of pathological shame is the fact that it leads to arrogance, self-deception, avoidance, and blaming of others. Such feelings may be bound up in the clinician's internal affective state or may be employed as a method in the training system itself. As a result, individual clinicians and professional groups develop a false sense of complacency that can lead to serious problems at both an individual and an organizational level. To learn something new, we must first acknowledge what we don't know. If we can stand to use them, self-assessment methods can assist us in this regard.

Choice of Training

Whether entering a residency program or seeking continuing education, it is important for every therapist to determine whether the training offered is coherent. The prestige of an institution is not an automatic guarantee. When evaluating a training program, it is possible to ask current students about the way that boundary issues are handled, and the mechanisms in place for dealing with problems concerning abusive faculty. Are faculty members generally respectful of students, or are they prone to use shaming? Every psychotherapy training program should have clearly thought-out and well-defined policies in this regard. Is there a policy for supervisors and teachers regarding the limits of personal involvement with students? Similarly, when seeking posttraining supervision, clinicians should find out as much as they can about a supervisor's ethical perspectives and approach to boundaries. A supervisor's fame as an academician does not ensure that he or she will be a good role model. On a collective scale, it would be helpful if prospective students asked more questions like these, because they would be likely to inspire training faculties to develop more sensitive and effective programs.

Personal Psychotherapy

When seeking personal psychotherapy as a supplement to training, clinicians should employ some of the same criteria used for finding a good supervisor. Personal therapy can assist an individual in exploring hidden or defensive motives for his or her career choice. Personal therapy should specifically include an effort to gain a better understanding of any fantasies or primary process expectations that are likely to be projected onto patients. Any motivation that goes beyond a desire to be involved in an interesting profession and to earn a good living might be problematic. Clinicians should be very cautious about staying with a personal therapist who has significant problems in maintaining boundaries. An example would be a therapist who becomes inordinately threatened when confronted with a minor boundary violation such as a lack of punctuality or a billing error. Such a therapist might provide an impaired model for the developing clinician, who is just learning to define his or her own therapeutic ego boundaries. Similarly, this type of personal therapist might be at higher risk of committing a major violation with the clinician-in-training that could be ruinous to his or her therapy and career.

Self-Assessment of Clinical Risk Factors

Many therapists are prone to diagnose and treat themselves. In so doing, they are at greater risk of having a biased observer, and they miss a timely opportunity to receive competent assistance. Self-help methods are often employed as a compulsive defense against pathological shame connected with feelings of weakness or vulnerability. The problem can become tragically intensified because some therapists refuse the very same help they are so ready to prescribe for others. Reluctance to seek personal care may be a sign that they are burdened by "rescue fantasies" (see Chapter 13). The following symptoms are key indicators that a therapist might use to alert himself or herself that a need exists to seek competent professional assistance.

Affective disorders.   If a therapist becomes aware that he or she is suffering from mood swings manifest by periods of elation, irritability, or depression; if any blood relatives have been treated for a mood disorder; or if colleagues, friends, or relatives question his or her judgment, that therapist should consider neuropsychiatric evaluation for a bipolar disorder. He or she may be in a high-risk group for committing serious boundary violations. Many talented and productive clinicians suffer from affective disorders. These therapists are usually able to function at a high level of competence with their patients if they obtain proper treatment for themselves.

Head trauma with associated personality changes.   If a therapist has suffered traumatic brain injury (TBI) from a blow to the cranium, and other persons observe a subsequent personality change or have reason to question that therapist's judgment, he or she should obtain consultation from a neuropsychiatrist or neuropsychologist specializing in TBI. Seemingly minor head trauma can lead to clinically significant behavioral problems, even when no loss of consciousness has occurred. A subclinical frontal lobe syndrome or other organic changes might be placing the therapist at high risk for using poor judgment with his or her patients. Positive evidence for impairment on neuropsychological testing does not necessarily mean that the therapist cannot continue practicing. A full evaluation will assist him or her to understand the nature and scope of any dysfunction, and may be invaluable in developing compensatory strategies and cognitive rehabilitation.

Grandiosity.   If a therapist starts to believe that he or she has developed special powers of healing that justify his or her being entitled to ignore the ordinary rules of behavior, that therapist is at very high risk of violating patients' boundaries. An antisocial variant of grandiosity is found in individuals who find it exhilarating to deceive or exploit other people, even when there may not be any material gain for them in such behavior. Lying for "sport" serves as an exciting way of feeling that one has obtained power over another person. Grandiosity is often a desperate defense against strong feelings of shame and vulnerability. Working on these issues with a psychotherapist might be very helpful in finding more adaptive and less dangerous ways of dealing with such feelings.

Substance abuse.   If a therapist's pattern of using alcohol or other drugs has led to family problems, missing work, loss of memory during drug or alcohol use (blackouts), driving while intoxicated, repeated unsuccessful efforts to cut down on intake, annoyance at friends and family over their attitude toward the drug or alcohol use, guilt over drinking or drug use, and/or using drugs or alcohol as a way of relaxing in the morning, or if the therapist uses substances such as amphetamines or cocaine, he or she should seek evaluation from a specialist in substance abuse disorders.

Sexual compulsions.   Even if a therapist reasons that his or her sexual feelings for a patient seem to fit a "normal" pattern, or that those feelings conform to the conventional stereotypes of romantic love, it is important for him or her to remember that patient-therapist sex is a perversion of a trust, just like incest. If the therapist's sexual desires feel overwhelming, he or she may be suffering from a paraphilia or "sexual addiction." A therapist who feels overpowered by such impulses toward patients and finds that he or she has trouble resisting them should consider seeking help from a colleague who treats sexual disorders. Advances in behavioral and pharmacological treatment of these conditions have improved the prognosis for recovery. Abel et al. (1992) have developed a cognitive-behavioral treatment that specifically addresses the impaired logic used by physicians who engage in sexual misconduct with patients. Although their approach was primarily designed to rehabilitate offenders under discipline by a professional licensing board, the same methods are likely to be effective with prodromal therapists who have not yet acted upon their fantasies. Some medications can relieve the internal pressure of inappropriate sexual urges without adversely affecting sexual performance in more normal social situations. For example, Kafka and Prentky (1992b) have found that fluoxetine was very helpful in relieving the compulsive urges of individuals suffering from paraphilias and nonparaphilic sexual addictions.

Continuing Education and Consultation

Formal training is the foundation of one's professional skills. However, it is dangerous to believe that completion of training is the end of learning and study. Because of the ambiguities and uncertainties inherent in the practice of psychotherapy, practitioners can easily become lulled into a false sense of security based on the idea that a familiar and habitual mode of operating is necessarily the best way. Therapists need to keep up with recent advances in clinical science by reading professional journals, discussing cases with trusted colleagues, and attending continuing education courses. Clinicians should obtain consultation from a respected colleague or from a peer supervision group if they find that they are having serious difficulties with a single patient, or if they notice that they are repeatedly experiencing the same problem with a number of different patients.

Self-Assessment Tests

It is important for clinicians to practice their self-assessment skills. A useful guiding principle for the therapist would be to maintain a healthy index of suspicion when he or she becomes too comfortable or complacent with his or her abilities. Such complacency may be a sign that the clinician's therapeutic ego boundaries are too closed to new information, or that he or she is more focused on a personal feeling of comfort than on what is happening with the patient. It may also be a precursor to being blind-sided by a clinical surprise. Self-assessment checklists can serve a useful function when a therapist becomes worried about clinical problems with one or more patients.

Menninger and Holzman (1973) developed a checklist of 21 items that can serve to alert psychotherapists to the fact that their modes of interaction with patients are being strongly influenced by pathological countertransferential impulses. I have paraphrased most of their items in Table 15–3.

Langs (1973) cautioned that patients will often "test" their therapists with an invitation to act out some unconscious theme that could sabotage the treatment. The underlying purpose is to determine if the therapist will be able to hold true to his or her therapeutic resolve, or failing that, to prove that he or she can be seduced into repeating the traumatically exploitive behaviors remembered from the patient's childhood. Typical behaviors cited by Langs included a patient's referring a friend to the therapist for treatment, asking the therapist to collude in deceiving an insurance company, offering the therapist expensive gifts, and failing to pay the fee in a timely fashion.

I developed the Exploitation Index (EI) in collaboration with Dr. Robert Simon (Epstein and Simon 1990) as a self-assessment test designed to help therapists evaluate their management of boundary issues. Derived from samples of various types of boundary violations collated from clinical examples and forensic cases, this instrument consists of 32 items that inquire about the frequency of behaviors, attitudes, and feelings manifested over the previous 2-year period with one's patients (see appendix). The EI can be used as form of self-consultation when another colleague is not readily available. It has been validated in a systematically sampled population of 532 psychiatrists (Epstein et al. 1992), and has a moderately high internal consistency (Cronbach's Alpha = .81). Each item is scored by frequency of occurrence, from 0 to 3. The total EI score can range from

Table 15–3. Partial summary of checklist designed by Menninger and Holzman (1973) to warn therapists when their feelings or behaviors may be signaling countertransference problems

- Recurrent erotic or affectionate feelings with patients.
- Laxness in dealing with patients who act out.
- Being too lax about late payment of the fee.
- Attempting to impress a patient.
- Attempting to impress peers about a patient's special qualities.
- Displaying a sadistic tone when offering an interpretation to a patient.
- Tardiness in starting sessions.
- Allowing sessions to run overtime in the absence of exigent clinical indications.
- Engaging in gossip about a patient with colleagues.
- Prematurely reassuring a patient as a way of alleviating one's own anxiety.
- Frequent drowsiness during sessions.
- Encouraging overdependence, such as offering a patient unneeded reassurance.
- Excessive fear about a patient's leaving treatment.
- A need to ask a patient to do favors.
- A need to repeatedly argue a point with a patient.

Source.   Adapted from Menninger and Holzman 1973, pp. 91–92.

0 to 96. Consistent with the findings of previous survey studies that inquired about patient-therapist sexual contact, women psychiatrists reported significantly lower EI scores on average (13.4 ± 7.3) than did men (16.4 ± 7.8). Psychiatrists who scored at a level of 27 or higher placed in the top 10% of the respondents surveyed. Although the EI does not inquire specifically about sexual *contact* with patients, factor analysis identified five items that, loaded together, indicate a tendency for some individuals to eroticize the treatment relationship (this "eroticism" factor was previously discussed in Chapter 12).

The Exploitation Index*

R ate yourself according to the frequency that the following statements reflect your behavior, thoughts, or feelings with regard to
any particular patients you have seen in psychotherapy *within the past
2 years*. Approximate frequency as follows:

Never (never engage in this activity):	0 points
Rarely (engage in this activity about once a year or less):	1 point
Sometimes (engage in this activity about once every 3 months):	2 points
Often (engage in this activity once a month or more):	3 points

1. Do you do any of the following for your family members or social
acquaintances: prescribing medication, making diagnoses, offering
psychodynamic explanations for their behavior?

2. Are you gratified by a sense of power when you are able to control
a patient's activity through advice, medication, or behavioral restraint (e.g., hospitalization, seclusion)?

3. Do you find the chronic silence or tardiness of a patient a satisfy-
ing way of getting paid for doing nothing?

---

*Reprinted from Epstein RS, Simon RI, Kay GG: Assessing boundary violations in
psychotherapy: survey results with the Exploitation Index. *Bull Menninger Clin*
56:150–166, 1992. Used with permission.

4. Do you accept gifts or bequests from patients?

5. Have you engaged in a personal relationship with a patient after treatment was terminated?

6. Do you touch your patients (exclude handshake)?

7. Do you ever use information learned from patients, such as business tips or political information, for your own financial or career gain?

8. Do you feel that you can obtain personal gratification by helping to develop your patient's great potential for fame or unusual achievement?

9. Do you feel a sense of excitement or longing when you think of a patient or anticipate her/his visit?

10. Do you make exceptions for your patients, such as providing special scheduling or reducing fees, because you find the patient attractive, appealing, or impressive?

11. Do you ask your patient to do personal favors for you (e.g., get you lunch, mail a letter)?

12. Do you and your patients address each other on a first-name basis?

13. Do you undertake business deals with patients?

14. Do you take great pride in the fact that such an attractive, wealthy, powerful, or important patient is seeking your help?

15. Have you accepted for treatment persons with whom you have had social involvement or whom you knew to be in your social or family sphere?

16. When your patient has been seductive with you, do you experience this as a gratifying sign of your own sex appeal?

17. Do you disclose sensational aspects of your patient's life to others (even when you are protecting the patient's identity)?

18. Do you accept a medium of exchange other than money for your services (e.g., work on your office or home, trading of professional services)?

19. Do you find yourself comparing the gratifying qualities you observe in a patient with the less gratifying qualities in your spouse or significant other (e.g., thinking: "Where have you been all my life?")?

20. Do you feel that your patient's problems would be immeasurably helped if only he/she had a positive romantic involvement with you?

21. Do you make exceptions in the conduct of treatment because you feel sorry for your patient, or because you believe that he/she is in such distress or so disturbed that you have no other choice?

22. Do you recommend treatment procedures or referrals that you do not believe to be necessarily in your patient's best interests, but that may be to your direct or indirect financial benefit?

23. Have you accepted for treatment individuals known to be referred by a current or former patient?

24. Do you make exceptions for your patient because you are afraid she/he will otherwise become extremely angry or self-destructive?

25. Do you take pleasure in romantic daydreams about a patient?

26. Do you fail to deal with the following patient behavior(s): paying the fee late, missing appointments on short notice and refusing to pay for the time (as agreed), seeking to extend the length of sessions?

27.   Do you tell patients personal things about yourself in order to impress them?

28.   Do you find yourself trying to influence your patients to support political causes or positions in which you have a personal interest?

29.   Do you seek social contact with patients outside of clinically scheduled visits?

30.   Do you find it painfully difficult to agree to a patient's desire to cut down on the frequency of therapy, or to work on termination?

31.   Do you find yourself talking about your own personal problems with a patient and expecting her/him to be sympathetic to you?

32.   Do you join in any activity with a patient that may serve to deceive a third party (e.g., an insurance company)?

References

Abel GG, Becker JV, Cunningham-Rathner J: Complications, consent and cognitions in sex between children and adults. Int J Law Psychiatry 7:89–103, 1984

Abel GG, Barrett DH, Gardos PS: Sexual misconduct by physicians. Journal of the Medical Association of Georgia 81:237–246, 1992

Ablow KR: Delicate business: money and therapy; payment colors the relationship between psychiatrist and patient. Psychiatric Times, August 1992, reprinted from the Washington Post

Adams F (tr): The Genuine Works of Hippocrates. New York, William Wood & Co, 1929, pp 278–280

Alexander J, Kolodziejski K, Sanville J, et al: On final terminations: consultation with a dying therapist. Clinical Social Work Journal 17:307–321, 1989

Alpher VS: Assessment of ego functioning in multiple personality disorder. J Pers Assess 56:373–387, 1991

American Academy of Psychiatry and the Law: Ethical Guidelines for the Practice of Forensic Psychiatry. Baltimore, MD, May 1987

American Psychiatric Association: Diagnostic and Statistical Manual of Mental Disorders, 3rd Edition, Revised. Washington, DC, American Psychiatric Association, 1987

American Psychiatric Association: The Principles of Medical Ethics With Annotations Especially Applicable to Psychiatry. Washington, DC, American Psychiatric Association, 1989

American Psychiatric Association: Fact Sheet: Patient/Therapist Sexual Contact. Washington, DC, American Psychiatric Association, April 1992

American Psychiatric Association: The Principles of Medical Ethics With Annotations Especially Applicable to Psychiatry. Washington, DC, American Psychiatric Association, 1993

American Psychological Association: Standard 4.07: Ethical Principles of Psychologists and Code of Conduct. American Psychologist, December 1992

Apfel RJ, Simon B: Patient-therapist sexual contact, I: psychodynamic perspectives on the causes and results. Psychother Psychosom 43:57–62, 1985

Apfel RJ, Simon B: Sexualized therapy: causes and consequences, in Sexual Exploitation of Patients by Health Professionals. Edited by Burgess AW, Hartman CR. New York, Praeger, 1986, pp 143–151

Appelbaum PS, Jorgenson L: Psychotherapist-patient sexual contact after termination of treatment: an analysis and a proposal. Am J Psychiatry 148:1466–1473, 1991

Appelbaum PS, Lidz CW, Meisel A: Informed Consent: Legal Theory and Clinical Practice. New York, Oxford University Press, 1987

Appelbaum SA: Evils in the private practice of psychotherapy. Bull Menninger Clin 56:141–149, 1992

Aquilina C: Violence by psychiatric inpatients. Med Sci Law 31:306–312, 1991

Arden M: Infinite sets and double binds. Int J Psychoanal 65:443–52, 1984

Aristotle: The Basic Works of Aristotle. Edited by McKeon R. New York, Random House, 1941

Armsworth MW: Qualitative analysis of adult incest survivors' responses to sexual involvement with therapists. Child Abuse Negl 14:541–554, 1990

Averill SC, Beale D, Benfer B, et al: Preventing staff-patient relationships. Bull Menninger Clin 53:384–393, 1989

Barnum RW: Informed consent for psychotherapy. Presented at the 23rd annual meeting of the American Academy of Psychiatry and the Law, Boston, MA, October 16, 1992

Bateson G: Minimal requirements for a theory of schizophrenia. Arch Gen Psychiatry 2:477–491, 1960

Bateson G, Jackson DJ, Haley J, et al: Toward a theory of schizophrenia. Behav Sci 1:251–264, 1956

Beck JC: Informed consent for psychotherapy. Presented at the 23rd annual meeting of the American Academy of Psychiatry and the Law, Boston, MA, October 16, 1992

Benson GL, Grunebaum J, Steisel S, et al: Curriculum subcommittee report. Working paper, December 1990. Presented at the Massachusetts House of Representatives Committee on Sexual Misconduct by Physicians, Therapists, and Other Health Professionals: Conference on training for treatment: how can it help? preventing sexual misconduct and the abuse of power by health care professionals through education. University of Massachusetts at Boston, MA, May 15, 1992

Bergler E: Psychopathology of ingratitude (1959), in Money and Emotional Conflicts. New York, International Universities Press, 1970, p 266

Berne E: Games People Play: The Psychology of Human Relationships. New York, Grove, 1964

Bion WR: Container and contained transformed: attention and interpretation (1970), in Seven Servants. New York, Jason Aronson, 1977, pp 106–124

Blackman P (ed): Mishnayoth Nezikin. New York, Judaica Press, 1965

Bleger J: Psychoanalysis of the psychoanalytic frame. Int J Psychoanal 48:511–519, 1966

Bloom JD: The character of danger in psychiatric practice: are the mentally ill dangerous? Bull Am Acad Psychiatry Law 17:241–255, 1989

Borys DS, Pope KS: Dual relationships between therapist and client: a national study of psychologists, psychiatrists, an social workers. Professional Psychology: Research and Practice 20:283–293, 1989

Bratter TE: Responsible therapeutic eros: the psychotherapist who cares enough to define and enforce behavior limits with potentially suicidal adolescents. Counseling Psychologist 5:97–104, 1975

Brodsky AH: Sex between patient and therapist: psychology's data and response, in Sexual Exploitation in Professional Relationships. Edited by Gabbard GO. Washington, DC, American Psychiatric Press, 1989, pp 15–25

Broucek FJ: Shame and its relationship to early narcissistic developments. Int J Psychoanal 63:369–378, 1982

Brown LS, Borys DS, Brodsky AM, et al: Psychotherapist-patient sexual contact after termination of treatment. Am J Psychiatry 149:979–980, 1992

Buber M: I and Thou, 2nd Edition. Translated by Smith RG. New York, Scribners, 1958 (original work published 1923)

Buie DH: The abandoned therapist. International Journal of Psychoanalytic Psychotherapy 9:227–231, 1982–1983

Burtt EA (ed): Dhammapada (the way of truth), in The Teachings of the Compassionate Buddha. New York, New American Library, 1955, p 65

Carr ML, Robinson GE, Stewart DE, et al: A survey of Canadian psychiatric residents regarding resident-educator sexual contact. Am J Psychiatry 148:216–220, 1991

Celenza A: Empathy, ego boundaries and deficits in the sense of self. Dissertation, Boston University, 1986

Celenza A: The misuse of countertransference love in sexual intimacies between therapists and patients. Psychoanalytic Psychology 8:501–509, 1991

Claman JM: Mirror hunger in the psychodynamics of sexually abusing therapists. Am J Psychoanal 47:35–40, 1987

Clifft MA: Writing about psychiatric patients. Bull Menninger Clin 50:511–524, 1986

Cobliner WG: The Geneva school of genetic psychology and psychoanalysis: parallels and counterparts, in The First Year of Life: A Psychoanalytic Study of Normal and Deviant Development of Object Relations. Edited by Spitz RA. New York, International Universities Press, 1965, pp 301–356

Cooper v National Railroad Passenger Corp et al, 45 Cal App 3d 389, 119 Cal Rptr 541, 1214 (1975). Citing Acosta v Southern Cal Rapid Transit Dist, 2 Cal 3d 19, 27 [84 Cal Rptr 184, 465 P2d 72]

Corcoran KJ: An exploratory investigation into self-other differentiation: empirical evidence for a monistic perspective on empathy. Psychotherapy, Research and Practice 19:63–68, 1982

American Medical Association Council on Ethical and Judicial Affairs: Conflicts of interest: physician ownership of medical facilities. JAMA 267:2366–2369, 1992

Crane TS: The problem of physician self-referral under the Medicare and Medicaid antikickback statute: the Hanlester Network case and the Safe Harbor regulation. JAMA 268:85–91, 1992

Dahlberg CC. Sexual contact between patient and therapist. Contemporary Psychoanalysis 6:107–124, 1970

Davis KL, Meara NM: So you think it is a secret. Journal for Specialists in Group Work 7:149–153, 1982

Daws D: Consent in child psychotherapy: the conflicts for child patients, parents and professionals. Journal of Child Psychotherapy 12:103–111, 1986

Dickstein E, Erlen J, Erlen JA: Ethical principles contained in currently professed medical oaths. Acad Med 66:622–624, 1991

Dietz PE, Warren JI: The sexually sadistic criminal: a case study. Presented at the 23rd Annual Meeting, American Academy of Psychiatry and the Law, Boston, MA, October 16, 1992

Doe J: A bibliography, 1545–1940, of the works of Ambrose Paré (1510–1590). Premier Chirugien & Conseiller du Roi. Amsterdam, Gerard Th. van Heusden, 1937 (first printing), reprinted 1976

Drellich MG: Money and countertransference, in Money and Mind. Edited by Klebanow S, Lowenkopf EL. New York, Plenum, 1991, pp 155–162

Dubovsky SL, Groban SE: Congenital absence of sensation. Psychoanal Study Child 30:49–73, 1975

Durkin HE: A systems approach to group therapy: theory and practice, in The Newer Therapies: A Sourcebook. New York, Van Nostrand Reinhold, 1982, pp 194–205

Dyer AR: Ethics and Psychiatry: Toward Professional Definition. Washington, DC, American Psychiatric Press, 1988

Elkind D: Piagetian psychology and the practice of child psychiatry. Journal of the American Academy of Child Psychiatry 21:435–445, 1982

Ende J, Kazis L, Ash A, et al: Measuring patients' desire for autonomy: decision making and information-seeking preferences among medical patients. J Gen Intern Med 4:23–30, 1989

Ende J, Kazis L, Moskowitz MA: Preferences for autonomy when patients are physicians. J Gen Intern Med 5:506–509, 1990

Epstein RS: Home nursing care as an adjunct to private outpatient psychotherapy. Bull Menninger Clin 46:445–457, 1982

Epstein RS: Posttraumatic stress disorder: a review of diagnostic and treatment issues. Psychiatric Annals 19:556–563, 1989

Epstein RS: Ganser syndrome, trance logic, and the question of malingering. Psychiatric Annals 21:238–244, 1991

Epstein RS: Avoidant symptoms cloaking the diagnosis of PTSD in patients with severe accidental injury. Journal of Traumatic Stress 6:451–458, 1993

Epstein RS, Janowsky DS: Research on the psychiatric ward: the effects on conflicting priorities. Arch Gen Psychiatry 21:455–463, 1969

Epstein RS, Simon RI: The Exploitation Index: an early warning indicator of boundary violations in psychotherapy. Bull Menninger Clin 54:450–465, 1990

Epstein RS, Simon RI, Kay GG: Assessing boundary violations in psychotherapy: survey results with the Exploitation Index. Bull Menninger Clin 56:150–166, 1992

Erickson MH, Rossi EL: Hypnotherapy: An Exploratory Casebook. New York, Irvington, 1979

Esman AH: Rescue fantasies. Psychoanal Q 56:263–270, 1987

Federn P: Ego Psychology and the Psychoses. New York, Basic Books, 1952

Feldman JL: The managed care setting and the patient-therapist relationship, in Managed Mental Health Care. Edited by Feldman JL, Fitzpatrick RJ. Washington, DC, American Psychiatric Press, 1992, pp 219–229

Feldman-Summers S, Jones G: Psychological impacts of sexual contact between therapists or other health care practitioners and their clients. J Consult Clin Psychol 52:1054–1061, 1984

Finell JS: Narcissistic problems in analysts. Int J Psychoanal 66:433–445, 1985

Finell JS: The merits and problems with the concept of projective identification. Psychoanal Rev 73:103–120, 1986

Forer BR: The therapeutic relationship: 1968. Paper presented at the annual meeting of the California State Psychological Association, Pasadena, CA, 1980

Frank JD, Frank JB: Persuasion and Healing: A Comparative Study of Psychotherapy, 3rd Edition. Baltimore, MD, Johns Hopkins University Press, 1991

Freinhar JP: Oedipus or Odysseus: developmental lines of narcissism. Psychiatric Annals 16:477–485, 1986

Freud S: The interpretation of dreams (1900), in The Standard Edition of the Complete Psychological Works of Sigmund Freud, Vol 5. Translated and edited by Strachey J. London, Hogarth Press, 1958, pp 1–338

Freud S: Jokes and their relation to the unconscious (1905), in The Standard Edition of the Complete Psychological Works of Sigmund Freud, Vol 8. Translated and edited by Strachey J. London, Hogarth Press, 1958, pp 9–258

Freud S: A special type of choice of object made by men: contributions to the psychology of love I. (1910), in The Standard Edition of the Complete Psychological Works of Sigmund Freud, Vol 11. Translated and edited by Strachey J. London, Hogarth Press, 1958, pp 165–175

Freud S: Recommendations to physicians practicing psychoanalysis (1912), in The Standard Edition of the Complete Psychological Works of Sigmund Freud, Vol 12. Translated and edited by Strachey J. London, Hogarth Press, 1958, pp 111–120

Freud S: On beginning the treatment: further recommendations on the technique of psychoanalysis (1913), in The Standard Edition of the Complete Psychological Works of Sigmund Freud, Vol 12. Translated and edited by Strachey J. London, Hogarth Press, 1958, pp 123–144

Freud S: Observations on transference-love: further recommendations on the technique of psycho-analysis III. (1915), in The Standard Edition of the Complete Psychological Works of Sigmund Freud, Vol 12. Translated and edited by Strachey J. London, Hogarth Press, 1958, pp 159–171

Freud S: Lines of advance in psycho-analytic therapy (1919), in The Standard Edition of the Complete Psychological Works of Sigmund Freud, Vol 17. Translated and edited by Strachey J. London, Hogarth Press, 1958, pp 159–168

Freud S: Beyond the pleasure principle (1920), in The Standard Edition of the Complete Psychological Works of Sigmund Freud, Vol 18. Translated and edited by Strachey J. London, Hogarth Press, 1958, pp 7–64

Gabbard GO, Pope KS: Sexual intimacies after termination: clinical, ethical, and legal aspects, in Sexual Exploitation in Professional Relationships. Edited by Gabbard GO. Washington, DC, American Psychiatric Press, 1989, pp 115–127

Gabbard GO: Psychodynamics of sexual boundary violations. Psychiatric Annals 21:651–655, 1991

Gabel S, Oster G, Pfeffer CR (eds): Difficult Moments in Child Psychotherapy. New York, Plenum, 1988

Gafner G, Trudeau V: Drawing the boundaries in staff-patient relationships. VA Practitioner 7:39–45, 1990

Galanter M: Network Therapy for addiction: a model for office practice. Am J Psychiatry 150:28–36, 1993

Ganser SJM: Zur lehre vom hysterischen daemmerzustande. (Toward the elucidation of the hysterical twilight state.) Archiv für Psychiatrie und Nervenkrankheiten 38:34–46, 1904

Gardner RA: Therapeutic Communication With Children: The Mutual Storytelling Technique. New York, Science House, 1971, pp 352–357

Gartrell N, Herman J, Olarte S, et al: Psychiatrist-patient sexual contact: results of a national survey, I: prevalence. Am J Psychiatry 143:1126–1131, 1986

Gartrell N, Herman J, Olarte S, et al: Psychiatric residents' sexual contact with educators and patients: results of a national survey. Am J Psychiatry 145:690–694, 1988

Geis G, Jesilow P, Pontell H, et al: Fraud and abuse of government medical benefit programs by psychiatrists. Am J Psychiatry 142:231–234, 1985a

Geis G, Pontell H, Keenan C, et al: Peculating psychologists: fraud and abuse against Medicaid. Professional Psychology: Research and Practice 16:823–832, 1985b

Glaser RD, Thorpe JS: A survey of sexual contact and advances between psychology educators and female graduate students. Am Psychol 41:43–51, 1986

Glassman MB: Intrapsychic conflict versus developmental deficit: a causal modeling approach to examining psychoanalytic theories of narcissism. Psychoanalytic Psychology 5:23–46, 1988

Goffman E: Frame Analysis: An Essay on the Organization of Experience. Cambridge, MA, Harvard University Press, 1974

Goldstein RL: When doctors divulge: is there a "threat from within" to psychiatric confidentiality? J Forensic Sci 34:433–438, 1989

Goldstein RL: Psychiatric poetic license? post-mortem disclosure of confidential information in the Anne Sexton case. Psychiatric Annals 22:341–348, 1992

Goldstein WN: Clarification of projective identification. Am J Psychiatry 148:153–161, 1991

Gonsiorek JC: Working therapeutically with therapists who have become sexually involved with their clients, in Psychotherapists' Sexual Involvement With Clients: Intervention and Prevention. Edited by Schoener GR, Milgrom JH, Gonsiorek JC, et al. Minneapolis, MN, Walk-In Counseling Center, 1990, pp 421–433

Gonsiorek JC, Brown LS: Post therapy sexual relationships with clients, in Psychotherapists' Sexual Involvement With Clients: Intervention and Prevention. Edited by Schoener GR, Milgrom JH, Gonsiorek JC, et al. Minneapolis, MN, Walk-In Counseling Center, 1990, pp 289–301

Gorton G, Samuel S: Prevention of therapist-patient sexual exploitation. Workshop presented at the 145th annual meeting of the American Psychiatric Association, Washington, DC, May 6, 1992

Greenfield S, Kaplan S, Ware JE: Expanding patient involvement in care: effects on patient outcomes. Ann Intern Med 102:520–528, 1985

Greenspan SI: The formation of the mind: implications for the prevention of autism and disorders of thought and affect. Lecture presented at the 145th annual meeting of the American Psychiatric Association, Washington, DC, May 6, 1992a

Greenspan SI: Infancy and Early Childhood: The Practice of Clinical Assessment and Intervention With Emotional and Developmental Challenges. Madison, CT, International Universities Press, 1992b

Greenspan SI, Curry JF: Piaget's approach to intellectual functioning, in Comprehensive Textbook of Psychiatry, 5th Edition, Vol 1. Edited by Kaplan HI, Sadock BJ. Baltimore, MD, Williams & Wilkins, 1989, pp 256–262

Gutheil TG: Borderline personality disorder, boundary violations, and patient-therapist sex: medicolegal pitfalls. Am J Psychiatry 146:597–602, 1989

Gutheil TG: Approaches to forensic assessment of false claims of sexual misconduct by therapists. Bull Am Acad Psychiatry Law 20:289–296, 1992

Gutheil TG, Gabbard GO: The concept of boundaries in clinical practice: theoretical and risk-management dimensions. Am J Psychiatry 150:188–196, 1993

Haley J: Strategies of Psychotherapy. Rockville, MD, Triangle, 1990

Harder DW: Character style of the defensively high self-esteem man. J Clin Psychol 40:26–35, 1984

Hartmann E: Boundaries in the Mind: A New Psychology of Personality. New York, Basic Books, 1991

Hartmann E, Russ D, Oldfield M, et al: Who has nightmares? the personality of the lifelong nightmare sufferer. Arch Gen Psychiatry 44:49–56, 1987

Herman JL: Complex PTSD: a syndrome in survivors of prolonged and repeated trauma. Journal of Traumatic Stress 5:377–391, 1992a

Herman JL: Trauma and Recovery. New York, Basic Books, 1992b, pp 87–88, 101–103

Hill L: Psychotherapeutic Intervention in Schizophrenia. Chicago, IL, University of Chicago Press, 1955

Holroyd JC, Brodsky AM: Psychologists' attitudes and practices regarding erotic and nonerotic physical contact with patients. Am Psychol 32:843–849, 1977

Holroyd JC, Brodsky AM: Does touching patients lead to sexual intercourse? Professional Psychology 11:807–811, 1980

Horner AJ: Money issues and analytic neutrality, in Money and Mind. Edited by Klebanow S, Lowenkopf EL. New York, Plenum, 1991, pp 175–181

Jackson JM, Stricker G: Supervision and the problem of grandiosity in novice therapists. Psychotherapy Patient 5:113–124, 1989

Jesilow P, Geis G, Pontell H: Fraud by physicians against Medicaid. JAMA 266:3318–3322, 1991

Johnson AM, Szurek SA: The genesis of antisocial acting out in children and adults. Psychoanal Q 21:323–343, 1952

Jones E: The Life and Work of Sigmund Freud, Vol 3. New York, Basic Books, 1957

Kafka MP, Prentky R: A comparative study of nonparaphilic sexual addictions and paraphilias in men. J Clin Psychiatry 53:345–350, 1992a

Kafka MP, Prentky R: Fluoxetine treatment of nonparaphilic sexual addictions and paraphilias in men. J Clin Psychiatry 53:351–358, 1992b

Karasu TB: The specificity versus nonspecificity dilemma: towards identifying therapeutic change agents. Am J Psychiatry 143:687–695, 1986

Kardener SH, Fuller M, Mensh IN: A survey of physicians' attitudes and practices regarding erotic and nonerotic contact with patients. Am J Psychiatry 130:1077–1081, 1973

Kearney M: Confidentiality in group psychotherapy. Psychotherapy in Private Practice 2:19–20, 1984

Kernberg OF: Borderline Conditions and Pathological Narcissism. New York, Jason Aronson, 1975

Klein M: Notes on some schizoid mechanisms. Int J Psychoanal 27:99–110, 1946

Kluft RP: Treating the patient who has been sexually exploited by a previous therapist. Psychiatr Clin North Am 12:483–500, 1989

Kluft RP: Paradigm exhaustion and paradigm shift: thinking through the therapeutic impasse. Psychiatric Annals 22:502–508, 1992

Kohut H: The Analysis of the Self: A Systematic Approach to the Psychoanalytic Treatment of Narcissistic Personality Disorders. New York, International Universities Press, 1971

Krueger DW: A self-psychological view of money, in The Last Taboo: Money as Symbol and Reality in Psychotherapy and Psychoanalysis. Edited by Krueger DW. New York, Brunner/Mazel, 1986, pp 24–32

Krystal H: Integration and Self-Healing: Affect, Trauma, Alexithymia. Hillsdale, NJ, Analytic Press, 1988

Landis B: Ego boundaries. Psychological Issues 4(4), Monograph 24, 1970

Langs R: The Technique of Psychoanalytic Psychotherapy, Vol 1. New York, Jason Aronson, 1973

Langs R: The framework of training analyses. International Journal of Psychoanalytic Psychotherapy 10:259–87, 1984–1985a

Langs R: Making interpretations and securing the frame: sources of danger for psychotherapists. International Journal of Psychoanalytic Psychotherapy 10:3–23, 1984–1985b

Lansky MR: Fathers Who Fail: Shame and Psychopathology in the Family System. Hillsdale, NJ, Analytic Press, 1992

Lanza ML, Carifio J: Blaming the victim: complex (nonlinear) patterns of causal attribution by nurses in response to vignettes of a patient assaulting a nurse. Journal of Emergency Nursing 17:299–309, 1991

La Puma J, Priest ER: Is there a doctor in the house? an analysis of the practice of physicians' treating their own families. JAMA 267:1810–1812, 1992

Lazare A: Expert shares advice on handling shame, humiliation in therapy. Psychiatric News, August 7, 1992, p 8

Lazarus JA, Sharfstein SS: APA acts against ethics violators. Psychiatric News, October 16, 1992, p 14

Leong GB, Silva JA, Weinstock R: Reporting dilemmas in psychiatric practice. Psychiatric Annals 22:482–486, 1992

Lerner H, Sugarman A, Barbour CG: Patterns of ego boundary disturbance in neurotic, borderline, and schizophrenic patients. Psychoanalytic Psychology 2:47–66, 1985

Levin R: Ego boundary impairment and thought disorder in frequent nightmare sufferers. Psychoanalytic Psychology 7:529–543, 1990

Lewis HB: Shame and Guilt in Neurosis. New York, International Universities Press, 1971

Lewis HB: Shame and the narcissistic personality, in The Many Faces of Shame. Edited by Nathanson DL. New York, Guilford, 1987, pp 93–132

Lidz CW, Meisel A, Zerubavel E, et al: Informed Consent: A Study of Decision Making in Psychiatry. New York, Guilford, 1984

Lion JR, Madden DJ, Christopher RL: A violence clinic: three years' experience. Am J Psychiatry 133:432–435, 1976

Luepker E: Sexual exploitation of clients by therapists: parallels with parent-child incest, in Psychotherapists' Sexual Involvement With Clients: Intervention and Prevention. Edited by Schoener GR, Milgrom JH, Gonsiorek JC, et al. Minneapolis, MN, Walk-In Counseling Center, 1990, pp 73–79

Madden DJ, Lion JR, Penna MW: Assaults on psychiatrists by patients. Am J Psychiatry 133:422–425, 1976

Maimonides M: Mishneh Torah. Annotated by Birnbaum P. New York, Hebrew Publishing, 1944, pp 21–22 [Hilchot De'ot 7], 237–238 [Hilchot Rotze'ach Ushmirat Nefesh 11]

Maimonides M: The Guide for the Perplexed. Translated by Friedlander M. New York, Dover, 1956

Mahler MS: On Human Symbiosis and the Vicissitudes of Individuation. New York, International Universities Press, 1968

Marks DF, Baird JM, McKellar P: Replication of trance logic using a modified experimental design: highly hypnotizable subjects in both real and simulator groups. Int J Clin Exp Hypn 37:232–248, 1989

Marmor J: Some psychodynamic aspects of the seduction of patients in psychotherapy. Am J Psychoanal 36:319–23, 1976

Maslow AH: Toward a Psychology of Being, 2nd Edition. New York, Van Nostrand Reinhold, 1968

Massachusetts House of Representatives Committee on Sexual Misconduct by Physicians, Therapists, and Other Health Professionals: Conference on training for treatment: how can it help? preventing sexual misconduct and the abuse of power by health care professionals through education. University of Massachusetts at Boston, MA, May 15, 1992

Matte-Blanco I: Expression in symbolic logic of the characteristics of the system ucs or the logic of the system ucs. Int J Psychoanal 40:1–5, 1959

Matte-Blanco I: Thinking, Feeling, and Being: Clinical Reflections on the Fundamental Antinomy of Human Beings and World. London, Routledge, 1988

Medlicott RW: Erotic professional indiscretions, actual or assumed and alleged. Aust N Z J Psychiatry 2:17–23, 1968

Menninger K, Holzman P: Theory of Psychoanalytic Technique, 2nd Edition. New York, Basic Books, 1973

Miller TR: The psychotherapeutic utility of the five-factor model of personality: a clinician's experience. J Pers Assess 57:415–433, 1991

Mitchell JM, Scott E: New evidence of the prevalence and scope of physician joint ventures. JAMA 268:80–84, 1992

Morrison AP: Shame, the ideal self, and narcissism. Contemporary Psychoanalysis 19: 295–318, 1983

Nathanson DL: A timetable for shame, in The Many Faces of Shame, Edited by Nathanson DL. New York, Guilford, 1987, pp 1–62

Nathanson DL: Shame and Pride: Affect, Sex, and the Birth of the Self. New York, Norton, 1992

O'Leary J, Wright F: Shame and gender issues in pathological narcissism. Psychoanalytic Psychology 3:327–340, 1986

Olness K, Gardner GG: Hypnosis and Hypnotherapy With Children. Philadelphia, PA, Grune & Stratton, 1988

Orne MT: The nature of hypnosis: artifact and essence. Journal of Abnormal and Social Psychology 58:277–299, 1959

Orne MT, Wender PH: Anticipatory socialization for psychotherapy: method and rationale. Am J Psychiatry 124:1202–1212, 1968

Palombo J: Critique of Schamess' concept of boundaries. Clinical Social Work Journal 15:284–293, 1987

Parker S: The precultural basis of the incest taboo: toward a biosocial theory. American Anthropologist 78:285–305, 1976

Parkes KR: Field dependence and the factor structure of the General Health Questionnaire in normal subjects. Br J Psychiatry 140:392–400, 1982

Perls FS: Gestalt Therapy Verbatim. Lafayette, CA, Real People Press, 1969

Perry JA: Physicians' erotic and nonerotic physical involvement with patients. Am J Psychiatry 133:838–840, 1976

Person ES: The erotic transference in men and women: differences and consequences. J Am Acad Psychoanal 13:159–180, 1985

Peterson MR: At Personal Risk: Boundary Violations in Professional-Client Relationships. New York, Norton, 1992

Piaget J: The stages of the intellectual development of the child. Bull Menninger Clin 26:120–128, 1962

Polster S: Ego boundary as process: a systemic-contextual approach. Psychiatry 46:247–258, 1983

Pope KS, Bouhoutsos JC: Sexual Intimacy Between Therapists and Patients. New York, Praeger, 1986

Pope KS, Vetter VA: Ethical dilemmas encountered by members of the American Psychological Association: a national survey. Am Psychol 47:397–411, 1992

Pope KS, Levenson H, Schover LR: Sexual intimacy in psychology training: results and implications of a national survey. Am Psychol 34:682–689, 1979

Pope KS, Keith-Spiegel P, Tabachnick BG: Sexual attraction to clients: the human therapist and the (sometimes) inhuman training system. Am Psychol 41:147–158, 1986

Porder M: Projective identification: an alternative hypothesis. Psychoanal Q 56:431–451, 1987

Racker H: The meanings and uses of countertransference. Psychoanal Q 26:303–357, 1957

Raynor E, Tuckett D: An introduction to Matte-Blanco's reformulation of the Freudian unconscious and his conceptualization of the internal world, in Matte-Blanco I, Thinking, Feeling, and Being: Clinical Reflections on the Fundamental Antinomy of Human Beings and World. London, Routledge, 1988, pp 3–42

Reid WH, Kang JS: Serious assaults by outpatients or former patients. Am J Psychother 40:594–600, 1986

Rhue JW, Lynn SJ: The use of hypnotic techniques with sexually abused children, in Clinical Hypnosis With Children. Edited by Wester WC, O'Grady DJ. New York, Brunner/Mazel, 1991, pp 69–84

Richman JA, Flaherty JA, Rospenda KM, et al: Mental health consequences and correlates of reported medical student abuse. JAMA 267:692–694, 1992

Roazen P: Brother Animal: The Story of Freud and Tausk. New York, Vintage Books, 1969

Rogers WH, Wells KB, Meredith LS, et al: Outcomes for adult outpatients with depression under prepaid or fee-for-service financing. Arch Gen Psychiatry 50:517–525, 1993

Roland A: Induced emotional reactions and attitudes. Psychoanal Rev 68:45–74, 1981

Rosenbloom S: The development of the work ego in the beginning analyst: thoughts on identity formation of the psychoanalyst. Int J Psycho-anal 73:117–126, 1992

Rosner F (tr): Maimonides' Mishneh Torah, Hilchot Rotze'ach 11:4, in Modern Medicine and Jewish Ethics. Hoboken, NJ, Ktav Publishing, 1986, pp 365–366 (For Hebrew text, see Maimonides 1944, pp 237–238)

Rosner F: The physician's prayer attributed to Moses Maimonides. Bull Hist Med 41:440–454, 1967

Rothstein A: The seduction of money, in Money and Mind. Edited by Klebanow S, Lowenkopf EL. New York, Plenum, 1991, pp 149–153

Rouse WHD (tr): Great Dialogues of Plato. New York, New American Library, 1956

Rubin HR, Gandek B, Rogers WH, et al: Patients' ratings of outpatient visits in different practice settings: results from the Medical Outcomes Study. JAMA 270:835–840, 1993

Rutter P: Sex in the Forbidden Zone. New York, Fawcett Crest, 1989

Saari C: Comments on Schamess' use of Langs' concept of the Frame. Clinical Social Work Journal 15:192–200, 1987

Schafer R: Aspects of internalization. New York, International Universities Press, 1968

Schneider CD: A mature sense of shame, in The Many Faces of Shame. Edited by Nathanson DL. New York, Guilford, 1987, pp 194–213

Schneider I: The theory and practice of movie psychiatry. Am J Psychiatry 144:996–1002, 1987

Schoener GR: A look at the literature, in Psychotherapists' Sexual Involvement With Clients: Intervention and Prevention. Edited by Schoener GR, Milgrom JH, Gonsiorek JC, et al. Minneapolis, MN, Walk-In Counseling Center, 1990, pp 11–50

Schoener GR, Gonsiorek JC: Assessment and development of rehabilitation plans for the therapist, in Psychotherapists' Sexual Involvement With Clients: Intervention and Prevention. Edited by Schoener GR, Milgrom JH, Gonsiorek JC, et al. Minneapolis, MN, Walk-In Counseling Center, 1990, pp 401–420

Schoener GR, Milgrom JH: False or misleading complaints, in Psychotherapists' Sexual Involvement With Clients: Intervention and Prevention. Edited by Schoener GR, Milgrom JH, Gonsiorek JC, et al. Minneapolis, MN, Walk-In Counseling Center, 1990, pp 147–155

Searles HF: Oedipal love in the countertransference (1959), in Collected Papers on Schizophrenia and Related Subjects. New York, International Universities Press, 1965, pp 284–303

Senior BA: Ego boundaries and the boundaries of tension systems. Dissertation, New School for Social Research, 1981

Shaw JA: Unmasking the illusion of safety: psychic trauma in war. Bull Menninger Clin 51:49–63, 1987

Sheehan KH, Sheehan DV, White K, et al: A pilot study of medical student "abuse": student perceptions of mistreatment and misconduct in medical school. JAMA 263:533–537, 1990

Shengold L: Soul murder: a review. International Journal of Psychoanalytic Psychotherapy 3:366–373, 1974

Shengold L: Anal erogeneity: the goose and the rat. Int J Psycho-anal 63:331–345, 1982

Shengold L: A variety of narcissistic pathology stemming from parental weakness. Psychoanal Q 60:86–92, 1991

Shor J, Sanville J: Erotic provocations and alliances in psychotherapeutic practice: some clinical cues for preventing and repairing therapist-patient collusions. Clinical Social Work Journal 2:83–95, 1974

Shuman DW: Current and future trends in PTSD litigation. Presented at the conference on The Development of Standards for the Forensic Examination of Post-Traumatic Stress Disorder Claimants. Georgetown University School of Medicine, Washington, DC, November 19, 1992

Siegel K: Anonymity. International Journal of Psychoanalytic Psychotherapy 11:183–218, 1985–1986

Silver HK, Glicken AD: Medical student abuse: incidence severity and significance. JAMA 263:527–532, 1990

Simon J: Integrity in the psychoanalytic relationship. Am J Psychoanal 49:77–85, 1989

Simon RI: The psychiatrist as a fiduciary: avoiding the double agent role. Psychiatric Annals 17:622–626, 1987

Simon RI: Sexual exploitation of patients. How it begins before it happens. Psychiatric Annals 19:104–112, 1989

Simon RI: Treatment boundary violations: clinical, ethical and legal considerations. Bull Am Acad Psychiatry Law 20:269–286, 1992a

Simon RI: Clinical Psychiatry and the Law, 2nd Edition. Washington, DC, American Psychiatric Press, 1992b

Slovenko R: Undue familiarity or undue damages? Psychiatric Annals 21:598–610, 1991

Spindler AC: Psychotherapist-patient sexual contact after termination of treatment. Am J Psychiatry 149:984–985, 1992

Spitz RA: The First Year of Life: A Psychoanalytic Study of Normal and Deviant Development of Object Relations. New York, International Universities Press, 1965, pp 138–143

Stone MH: Management of unethical behavior in a psychiatric hospital staff. Am J Psychother 29:391–401, 1975

Stone MH: Boundary violations between therapist and patient. Psychiatric Annals 6:670–677, 1976

Styron W: Sophie's Choice. New York, Random House, 1976, pp 481–487

Sugg NK, Inui T: Primary care physicians' response to domestic violence: opening Pandora's box. JAMA 267:3157–3160, 1992

Summit RC: The child sexual abuse accommodation syndrome. Child Abuse Negl 7:177–193, 1983

Szasz T: The problem of privacy in training analysis: selections from a questionnaire study of psychoanalytic practices and opinions. Psychiatry 25:195–207, 1962

Szekacs J: Impaired spatial structures. Int J Psychoanal 66:193–199, 1985

Tabachnick BG, Keith-Spiegel P, Pope KS: Ethics of teaching: beliefs and behaviors of psychologists as educators. Am Psychol 46:506–515, 1991

Tabin JK: Transitional objects as objectifiers of the self in toddlers and adolescents. Bull Menninger Clin 56:209–220, 1992

Talan KH: Gifts in psychoanalysis: theoretical and technical issues. Psychoanal Study Child 44:149–63, 1989

Tanke ED, Yesavage JA: Characteristics of assaultive patients who do and do not provide visible cues of potential violence. Am J Psychiatry 142:1409–1413, 1985

Tannen D: You Just Don't Understand: Women and Men in Conversation. New York, Morrow, 1990

Tarasoff v Regents of the University of California, 17 Cal 3d 425, 131 Cal Rptr 14, 551 P2d 334 (1976)

Tausk V: On the origin of the "Influencing Machine" in schizophrenia (1918) (translated by Feigenbaum D). Psychoanal Q 2:519–556, 1933 [Reprinted in Journal of Psychotherapy Practice and Research 1:184–206, 1992]

Terr L: Chowchilla revisited: the effects of psychic trauma four years after a school-bus kidnapping. Am J Psychiatry 140:1543–1550, 1983

Tolpin M: On the beginnings of a cohesive self: an application of the concept of transmuting internalization to the study of the transitional object and signal anxiety, in The Psychoanalytic Study of the Child, Vol 26. New York, Quadrangle Books, 1972, pp 313–352

Tomkins SS: Shame, in The Many Faces of Shame. Edited by Nathanson DL. New York, Guilford, 1987, pp 133–161

Tulipan AB: Fee policy as an extension of the therapist's style and orientation, in The Last Taboo: Money as Symbol and Reality in Psychotherapy and Psychoanalysis. Edited by Krueger DW. New York, Brunner/Mazel, 1986, pp 79–87

Twemlow SW, Gabbard GO: The lovesick therapist, in Sexual Exploitation in Professional Relationships. Edited by Gabbard GO. Washington, DC, American Psychiatric Press, 1989, pp 71–87

Uchill AB: Deviation from confidentiality and the therapeutic holding environment. International Journal of Psychoanalytic Psychotherapy 7:208–219, 1978–1979

Ulman RB, Brothers D: The Shattered Self: A Psychoanalytic Study of Trauma. Hillsdale, NJ, Analytic Press, 1988

United States Tennis Association: Friend at Court: Rules of Tennis. New York, USTA, 1992, pp 4–23

van Mens-Verhulst J: Perspective of power in the therapeutic relationship. Am J Psychother 45:198–210, 1991

Viderman S: Interpretation in the analytic space. International Review of Psycho-Analysis 1:467–480, 1974 von Bertalanffy L: General Systems Theory. New York, Braziller, 1968

Wachtel TJ, Stein MD: Fee-for-time system: a conceptual framework for an incentive-neutral method of physician payment. JAMA 270:1226–1229, 1993

Watkins HH: Ego-state therapy: an overview. Am J Clin Hypn 35:232–240, 1993

Watkins JG, Watkins HH: Ego-state therapy, in The Newer Therapies: A Sourcebook. New York, Van Nostrand Reinhold, 1982, pp 136–155

Watkins JG, Watkins HH: The management of malevolent ego states in multiple personality disorder. Dissociation 1:67–72, 1988

Watkins JG, Watkins HH: Dissociation and displacement: where goes the "ouch?" Am J Clin Hypn 33:1–21, 1990

Webb WL: The doctor-patient covenant and the threat of exploitation. Am J Psychiatry 143:1149–1150, 1986

Welt SR, Herron WG: Narcissism and the Psychotherapist. New York, Guilford, 1990

Wheelis A: The Doctor of Desire. New York, WW Norton, 1987

Whitman RM, Bloch EL: Therapist envy. Bull Menninger Clin 54:478–487, 1990

Whitman RM, Armao BB, Dent OB: Assault on the therapist. Am J Psychiatry 133:426–429, 1976

Winchell C: It's O.K. to prescribe for friends and family but . . . Montgomery Medicine 38:17, 1992

Winnicott DW: Transitional objects and transitional phenomena (1951), in Collected Papers: Through Paediatrics to Psycho-analysis. New York, Basic Books, 1958, pp 229–242

Winnicott DW: Counter-transference (1960a), in The Maturational Processes and the Facilitating Environment: Studies in the Theory of Emotional Development. New York, International Universities Press, 1965, pp 158–165

Winnicott DW: Ego distortion in terms of true and false self (1960b), in The Maturational Processes and the Facilitating Environment: Studies in the Theory of Emotional Development. New York, International Universities Press, 1965, pp 140–152

Winnicott DW: The theory of the parent-infant relationship
(1960c), in The Maturational Processes and the Facilitating Environment: Studies in the Theory of Emotional Development.
New York, International Universities Press, 1965, pp 37–55

Winnicott DW: A personal view of the Kleinian contribution
(1962), in The Maturational Processes and the Facilitating Environment: Studies in the Theory of Emotional Development. New
York, International Universities Press, 1965, pp 171–178

Winnicott DW: Dependence in infant-care, in child-care, and in the
psycho-analytic setting (1963), in The Maturational Processes
and the Facilitating Environment: Studies in the Theory of Emotional Development. New York, International Universities Press,
1965, pp 249–259

Wurmser L: Shame: the veiled companion of narcissism, in The
Many Faces of Shame. Edited by Nathanson DL. New York,
Guilford, 1987, pp 64–92

Wynne LC, Ryckoff IM, Day J, et al: Pseudomutuality in the family
relations of schizophrenia. Psychiatry 21:205–220, 1958

Yalom ID: The Theory and Practice of Group Psychotherapy. New
York, Basic Books, 1970

Yalom ID, Lieberman MA: A study of encounter group casualties.
Arch Gen Psychiatry 25:16–30, 1971

Zinner J, Shapiro R: Projective identification as a mode of perception
and behavior in families of adolescents. Int J Psychoanal 53:523–
530, 1972

Index

*Page numbers printed in **boldface** type refer to tables or figures.*